SAD DOG
HAPPY DOG

How Poor Posture
Affects Your Child's Health

&

What You Can
Do About It

KATHLEEN PORTER

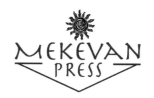

MEKEVAN PRESS

Mekevan Press
P.O. Box 393
Pepeʻekeo, HI 96785

Library of Congress Cataloging-in-Publication Data
Porter, Kathleen, 1947-
  Sad dog happy dog : how poor posture affects your child's health and what you can do about it / Kathleen Porter.

ISBN-978-0-615-37853-4

Library of Congress Control Number 2010909929

To the children:

May you always know yourselves to be a part of, not apart from, Nature. Herein lies hope for ourselves and our planet.

Table of Contents

Foreword

Introduction

Part 1   The Unrecognized Epidemic

One   In the Beginning: What Babies Teach Us

Two   Why Natural Alignment Matters

Three   Keeping Children Naturally Aligned

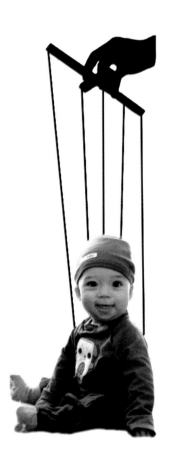

Part II Puppet Power — Guidelines & Instructions

FOREWORD

It is a pleasure to offer this commentary on my dear friend Kathleen Porter's book, *Sad Dog, Happy Dog,* that addresses skeletal alignment and spinal health. My personal journey with this started when my sister Trace and I opted to take a workshop on skeletal alignment taught by Kathleen at the Omega Institute in Rhinebeck, New York. During the course of the week-long class, we learned how to sit, stand, bend, walk and sleep comfortably, while also learning the ABCs of the biomechanics of the human design. This natural alignment has never been lost in some people who live in places where human labor dominates. In modern life and technology-oriented Western cultures, unnatural skeletal alignment has resulted in spinal impairment that creates the basis for unhealthy living.

Kathleen was truly an inspiration in helping us learn and grow within our bodies. We learned to laugh, share, and correct our mistakes while we reshaped our bodies. We started to reconstruct our spines into those of healthy adults, just as babies do naturally from birth. *Sad Dog, Happy Dog* is sure to become a classic in helping children and adults learn healthy spinal habits as they journey through life. I am honored and privileged to recommend this book to others who seek health and want to be able to live life fully!

John W. Metcalf, Ph.D., M.D.

INTRODUCTION

This book is the "missing manual" that addresses the slouching epidemic plaguing millions of children, as well as their parents and teachers. Forget what you've always believed about good posture being hard work; this book presents all new information on how to achieve relaxed, easy posture, while making for a fun adventure in mutual learning that adults and children can embark on together. Learning to find the support of aligned bones is the key to easy, relaxed posture that does not require the effort of straining, struggling muscles to pull us up or hold us together. Using this book as a guide, and their own bodies as personal laboratories for conducting simple explorations done together, adults and children can re-learn what every healthy toddler first discovers when learning how to stand and walk.

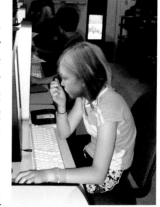

Children today are in trouble. The health-compromising changes that have taken hold in their bodies in recent generations have occurred gradually enough that, as a society, we have adapted our perceptions, much like the unsuspecting frog in a pot of slowly heating water. We have missed recognizing the seriousness of the growing physical melt-down many children face today.

Most of us know on some level that our children's poor posture is a problem. We struggle to know what to do about it, having learned first-hand the futility of telling a child to "sit up straight." Every day, frustrated teachers look out across classrooms filled with collapsed bodies and have to wonder at their students' ability to fully engage with the lesson at hand. Even when children do try to do as we ask, they misunderstand what natural posture actually is. They've been taught, as we have, to lift their chests skyward, using tension to keep themselves there. Without the support of aligned bones, however, they inevitably sink back down into the same familiar heap. Were we to fully understand the long-term consequences of chronically poor posture on our children's future health, we ourselves would "sit up straight" with alarm.

Many parents and teachers are at a loss to know how to inhabit their own bodies in ways that are comfortable and relaxed, yet strong and energetic. Can we ever expect children to listen to us if we don't know how to model better posture ourselves? How often do we demonstrate to our children that we are aware of our connection to the natural world? In the same way that a monkey is unlikely to throw out its shoulder while swinging from a tree, and a cheetah doesn't strain its hips or back from simply running fast, those humans who have not lost the natural alignment they first discovered as toddlers do not suffer from back or joint pain, even if they engage in what is often thought of today as "hard" labor. Almost any physical activity, even carrying a heavy bucket of water on one's head,

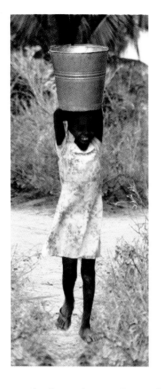

as the small child pictured here is doing, can be done with remarkable comfort and ease when bones are aligned. When one is not aligned, such an activity can, and often does, result in strain, discomfort and possibly injury.

I hope that we are on the verge of recognizing how important the alignment of our bones is to overall health and wellbeing. The fact that these details are overlooked in such a nearly universal manner is a reflection of just how disconnected modern-day humans have become from our roots in the natural world. We ignore this disconnection at our peril. We've lost sight of the fact that for all of humanity's remarkable and unique qualities, we are, as physical beings, still creatures of nature. In recent years, we have come to understand the relationship between good health and a diet that is based on natural, unprocessed food. One can only hope that our eyes will soon open to the relationship between good health and the natural body—not the "sculpted," unnatural and contrived one created by a gym workout or one made lean by a dependence on stretching exercises in order to feel free of tension—but one that upholds the easy flexibility, bone-deep strength and enduring vitality that is the birthright of anyone who is fortunate enough to be born healthy. Governed by the same natural laws that apply to physics, engineering and all things material, modern humans have traveled away from our own physical connection to the natural world. The further we stray from our natural design, the more likely we are to suffer back, neck and joint pain, along with a host of related health problems not experienced by those people in the world who still live according to nature's laws. Today, the incidence of injuries and idiopathic or "non-specific" pain among children in technologically advanced places is growing at an alarming rate, while continuing to be a growing epidemic among adults, as well.

The inspiration for this book grew out of my work with fourth-grade public school students in Hilo, Hawai`i. After spending a number of years coaching adults in how to align their bones for greater ease of movement and relief from pain, I became interested in knowing if children were good candidates for learning this. They were, after all, only a few years past their own early discovery of how to align their skeleton along its vertical axis, in order to be able to sit up, stand, and walk. Every healthy baby discovers this on its own, an act which is humanity's most direct connection to the earth we call home. Even at their tender age, many of the fourth graders I met were already in a state of chronic structural collapse. When questioned, many of them reported aching backs, neck pain and problems with sleeping.

I started out to teach the children, but they ended up teaching me. They taught me that they are hungry to know about themselves, that they respond with enthusiasm when they are encouraged to experience and *feel* what it means to *be*

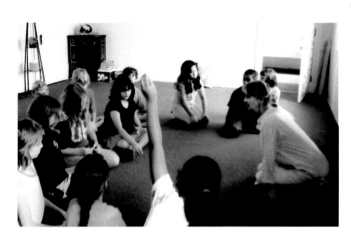

a body. They showed me that they are innately intelligent and have good instincts and that they have no difficulty embracing these concepts, *as long as adults are willing to do the same.* "Walk your talk" and "practice what you preach" are the actions that determine what kind of influence, if any, we will have on children's behavior.

Children are willing to accept our wisdom and authority, but make no mistake: They see very clearly when we are being hypocritical and setting a different standard for them than we set for ourselves. They respect us when we show a willingness to be open to learning new things about ourselves, and they recognize the value of something when we demonstrate our own belief in its importance. And, finally, they thrive with enthusiasm when they are included as equal partners in an adventure of self-discovery.

By the age of nine or ten, most children can easily comprehend the fundamentals of skeletal alignment, as well as concepts such as gravity and verticality. They have no difficulty understanding this information when it is conveyed in an experiential, personally relevant way. Although applying these concepts to one's daily life requires a level of self-awareness that can be fleeting in most children, particularly when they are bombarded with endless stimulation in their environment, the fact that children are becoming more "self-conscious" at this age is an asset in their developing ability to grasp these ideas. This approach has shown to be highly successful because it is both meaningful and *fun*. Adult participation is the key to this program's success, and for this reason, it is essential that parents and teachers involve themselves in improving their own posture as equal partners in a process of mutual learning with their children.

I thank the children I've worked with for forcing me to simplify the instructions I had been using for a number of years. This led to the creation of the *Puppet Posture* approach, as well as the *Sad Dog, Happy Dog* concept that helps make s easy sense of how a pelvis can move or "tilt". This is a crucial point, because the position of the pelvis determines the angle of the platform on which the spine sits. It's not unusual for children, especially in a group situation, to be overcome by nervous laughter at the mere mention of certain body parts such as "pelvis" or "pubic" bone. Yet, asking them to imagine that they are a little dog who is being scolded for chewing a slipper gives them an easily accessible way to experience the backward pelvic tilt of a "Sad Dog" tucking its tail between its legs. In contrast, a "Happy Dog" doesn't tuck its tail under, it wags its tail behind. With just a little more information about the rib cage, children are able to readily understand the relationship of the pelvis to the spine. Once children are involved with these ideas, any initial embarrassment disappears quickly, making it easier to introduce anatomical details without an outbreak of nervous silliness.

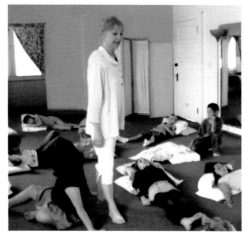

Cultivating awareness is a challenge for anyone, at any age, but this approach offers specific, concrete tools for being anchored in the present. Because changing our habits is ultimately an "inside job" that can never be accomplished for us by someone else, this approach helps children learn valuable lessons about paying attention to themselves—being mindful—while getting to know themselves inside their skin. In time, they become less self-conscious in ways that emphasize separation from others and more Self-conscious in ways that remind them of their connection with the world around them and the people in it.

The adults in children's lives have many opportunities to guide children toward a healthy future. Rather than simply telling kids to sit or stand "up straight", adults must first understand what this really means and then teach by example. They can also work to support very young children in never losing natural alignment in the first place and creating conditions that help older children learn how to return to "home base". Sports coaches can model and teach ways to move and participate in sports that are in keeping with the body's design, rather than letting poor habits of use become more deeply entrenched in the musculature through the repetitive movements of physical activity. Structural misalignment may contribute, more than anything else, to the current rise in the number of sports-related injuries among children. Pediatricians and other physicians can help children by taking into account a child's underlying skeletal structure as being an important aspect of a symmetrical and integrated whole that is important to the healthy functioning of all of the body's systems. Teachers can play a key role by incorporating these tools into the daily lesson and classroom activities. Parents can provide their children with alternatives to sitting in a crumpled heap in front of the television or computer screen, taking the time to make sure healthy options for sitting are available. Parents of infants and toddlers can be conscious of helping their children remain natural, so that they don't lose their essential alignment in the first place. The key point here is that it is not only what activities we do but how we do them that matters. With this book in hand, parents and teachers, sports coaches and health professionals will have tools for knowing what to do.

This book is divided into two distinct parts. Part One makes the case for natural alignment, detailing what it is and why it matters so much. This section is directed toward adults, although many children will enjoy going through this section, as well. Follow a child's lead if he or she shows interest in knowing more. Part Two is for adults and children to use together. Children will still need plenty of adult input when going through these pages, referring to the images, as parents and teachers interpret the written instructions. While these instructions may seem complex at first, they will become more clear and understandable as you move through and experiment with them. Expanded instructions and information are included on some facing pages for those who want to delve more deeply into the why of the instructions. Guidelines for walking have been greatly simplified in order to help break out of habitual patterns by getting out of the "thinking mind" and into the "moving mind". Step-by-step instructions for how to move through space can be hopelessly complicated, but by learning to surrender to the gentle "pull of the puppeteer", we can allow our bodies to be drawn through space in a way that is fluid and free.

I will end this with a brief story of how I decided to write this book. Some months after the conclusion of the initial pilot project in Hawaii, I had a conversation with Kathy Wines, the fourth grade teacher who personified all the best qualities of a nurturing, enthusiastic role model for her students. She found it helpful to be able to remind her students when she saw "Sad Dogs" in the room, as this served as a simple reminder for them to, first and foremost, arrange the pelvis as the foundation for easy upright sitting. One day, sometime after the program had ended, when Kathy again reminded the class that she saw some "Sad Dogs" in the room, one boy blurted out, "That's over!" My heart sank momentarily as Kathy told me this, before she added that another child called out, "No it's not! It's your whole life!"

Working with children in any capacity is always about planting seeds. Inspiring interest is the first step, because enthusiasm is the fertile soil in which the seeds can sprout. Our own enthusiasm for learning how to align our own bones is contagious. In the months and years ahead, the seeds sprout and grow, as long as they are nurtured by encouraging adults who are working in a light-hearted way to model this way of inhabiting their own bodies. As the sprouted seeds eventually grow to bear fruit, our children will reap the benefits for a whole lifetime. We will have helped to protect their—and our own—health by demonstrating how to avoid unnecessary pain and tension, providing tools for cultivating mindfulness and insured that they will enjoy authentic strength, easy flexibility and enduring vitality throughout a healthy lifetime.

PART I

The Unrecognized Epidemic

ONE

In the Beginning

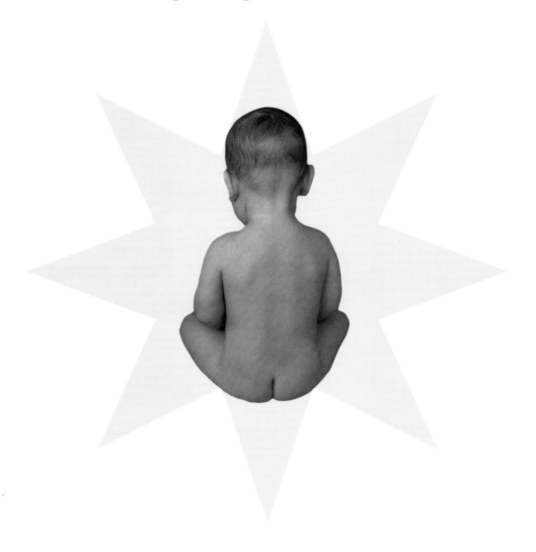

Healthy babies come into the world with the potential to live a lifetime of solid uprightness, enduring physical comfort and great ease of movement.

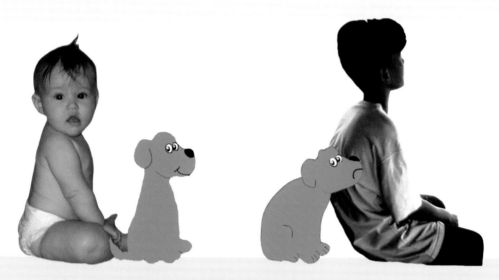

It doesn't take long for many children to develop chronic, health-damaging collapse. This problem has been growing progressively worse with successive generations. Those parents, teachers and health professionals who are aware of this problem are often at a loss to know what to do about it.

- This baby sits comfortably without strain or effort.

- Naturally aligned bones provide her with the support she needs to be upright.

- Her spine is straight, long and open. There is no pressure on spinal nerves.

- Her diaphragm is elastic and aids in free, relaxed breathing.

- Ample space in her torso provides for efficient functioning of vital organs.

- Good circulation of blood, lymphatic fluids and enzymes through an assortment of vessels, valves and "tubes" contributes to good health.

- If she never loses this alignment, this child is likely to enjoy generally good health.

- This boy sits in a state of constant collapse.

- He gets no support from misaligned bones.

- His spine is severely compressed, limiting optimal flow of impulses through the spinal cord and all the nerves that run through it.

- His diaphragm is distorted and frozen; relaxed breathing is impossible.

- His organs are compressed, impairing their efficient functioning.

- Circulation of blood and fluids is severely impaired.

- His bones are still forming, creating potentially serious problems in the future.

Each of these children is supported by a skeleton that is aligned along a center line, the vertical axis of gravity.

Their muscles are free of excess tension.

Their joints are flexible.

Once they master standing and walking, they move with ease, adhering to the natural human mechanical design.

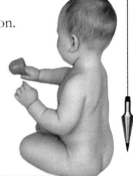

Babies and toddlers hold the secret of how to live in bodies that are naturally flexible, genuinely strong and free of aches and pains.

The **vertical axis of gravity** around which the skeleton is organized is the same **"plumb line"** to which builders refer when constructing a building.

Babies learn to sit up by balancing a bowling ball (the head) on top of a stick (the spine) through a focused process of concentration and surrender, much like learning to ride a bicycle. With practice, they find a delicate balance point—the vertical axis of gravity—that is the center line that governs everything in our physical world.

Healthy babies have at least one thing in common with happy dogs: they "wag their tails behind them". When a baby is able to balance upright, it is because she or he has found the position of the pelvis that supports a fully lengthened spine with the head balanced on top.

Sitting this way, a baby is grounded on a tripod of support between three points of the pelvis: the pubic bone and the front edge of the "sit bones" (sometimes referred to as the "sitz" bones and formally called the *ischial tuberosities*).

Happy Dog Pelvis
"Wagging Tail Pelvis"

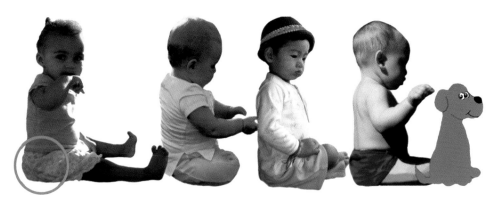

Healthy babies discover the natural position of the pelvis that offers a lifetime of easy, comfortable uprightness.

The natural position of the pelvis establishes the correct foundation for the spine, which, in turn, supports the torso and head.

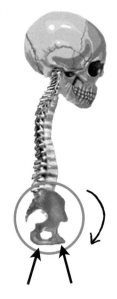

The babies pictured above have learned how to balance upright by letting their weight drop down onto the front of the pelvis or the pubic bone (*pubis ramus*). This is the position that allows them to discover the vertical axis of gravity within themselves. In this position the pelvis is anteverted or tipped forward. One way to remember this is to imagine the pelvis as a bowl filled with water. In this position, all the water would be poured out the front of the bowl.

Sit bones *Pubis ramus*

• Toddlers' muscles are relaxed, with just enough tone and elasticity to support an aligned, upright skeleton.

• An aligned skeleton is the framework of support for all of the body's systems.

• Babies are role models for the natural, healthy use of the body. They have not yet taken on poor habits of use or had unnatural patterns embedded in their musculature due to falls, injury or poor habits.

Sad Dog Pelvis

"Tucked Tail Pelvis"

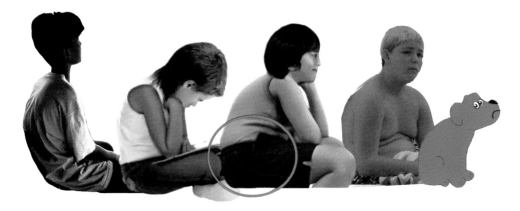

Within just a few years, most children today lose the support of aligned bones.

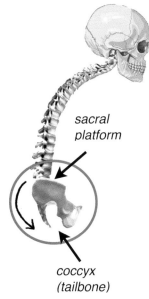

sacral platform

coccyx (tailbone)

A "tucked under" tailbone (*coccyx*) disrupts the angle of the sacral platform on which the spine sits, causing the spine to collapse and round.

When the weight of the spine and the head that rests on top of it are forced down onto the back edge of the sit bones, the spine is no longer able to align along the central axis and cannot distribute the forces of gravity through a vertical line.

•   We often think of collapsing as "letting go" and relaxing, but without the support of aligned bones, many muscles are put under tremendous stress and are anything but relaxed.

•   Without an aligned skeletal framework of support for all of the body's systems, those systems are also put under stress, as is the spine itself, the front of which is compressed .

•   The best remedy is always prevention of skeletal collapse in the first place.

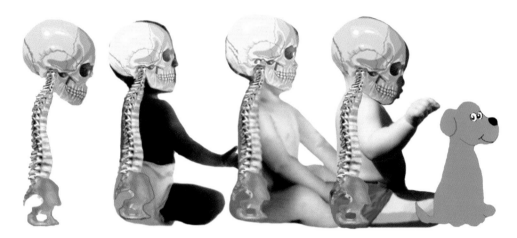

All aligned spines are the same, with vertebrae and intervertebral discs stacked directly one on top of the other. This allows the spine to be a mostly self-supporting structure, with only a minimum of muscular tension involved in being upright. Spinal curves are most evident through the vertebral column, the weight-bearing part of the spine. Curves are less pronounced through the spinous and transverse processes, the back of the spine where the facets, or joints, are located.

When babies discover the central axis, they are able to successfully balance a heavy head, poised delicately on top of the spine.

As seen in the examples below, this upright human design can remain intact well into adulthood and old age.

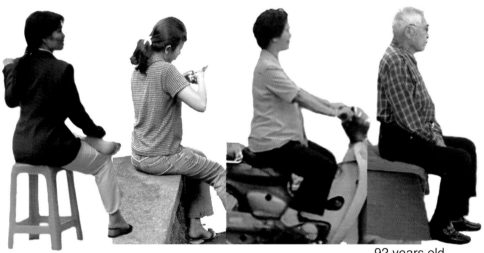

92 years old

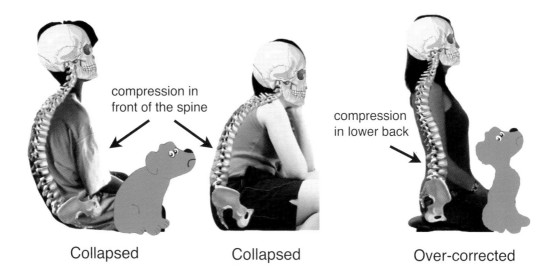

compression in
front of the spine

compression
in lower back

Collapsed   Collapsed   Over-corrected

Trying to sit up straight often results in over-correcting (far right). This lifting of the chest causes the lower back to arch, putting pressure on intervertebral discs, while holding muscles in constant contraction.

All the postures pictured here, whether collapsed or over-corrected, are at the root of most chronic back pain experienced by millions of people today. Many common conditions of the spine such as herniated or "bulging" discs, osteoarthritis, "degenerative disc disease" and spinal stenosis are likely to be caused by chronic misalignment of the skeleton. Aging looks and feels different for anyone who has lived in a state of chronic collapse.

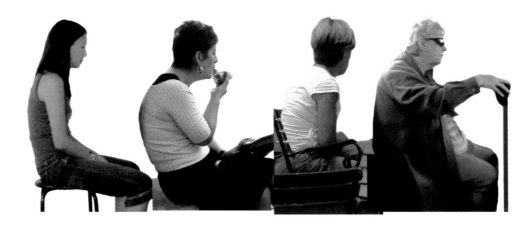

Children once sat on an aligned pelvis that supported an open spine.

It's easy to confuse greater formality of dress and lifestyle with rigidity and stiffness, but these children are supported by aligned bones, and their muscles are actually relaxed. They did not have to be told to "sit up straight" since, for them, doing so is "normal."

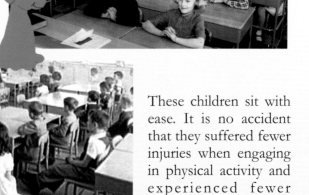

These children sit with ease. It is no accident that they suffered fewer injuries when engaging in physical activity and experienced fewer health problems. While the importance of a healthy diet is widely understood, the necessity of aligned bones is generally ignored.

Most children in America today have lost the support of aligned bones.

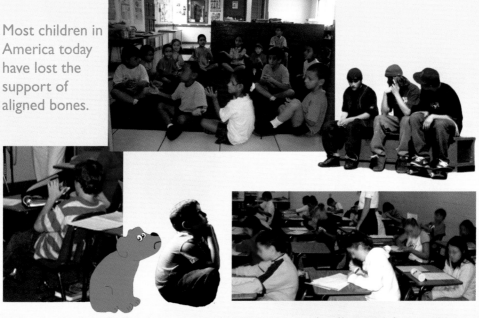

The "tucked under" pelvis causes chronic structural collapse and may play a large role in causing many more children today to complain of what doctors call "unexplained pain".

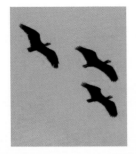
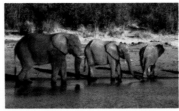
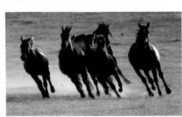
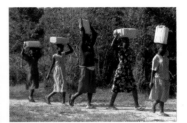

Nature's Rules

Every species in nature has a mechanical design that is particular to that species' needs. Vertebrates are those species that have backbones, or spinal columns, as well as a system of pulleys (muscles) and levers (bones) that adhere to the same physical laws that apply to everything else in our world, including physics and engineering.

The primary job of bones is to provide a solid framework of support for all the parts of the body. While muscles do, in some instances, provide support for this framework, their main job is to move the bones, not to hold us up. All healthy babies discover these laws when learning how to stand and walk.

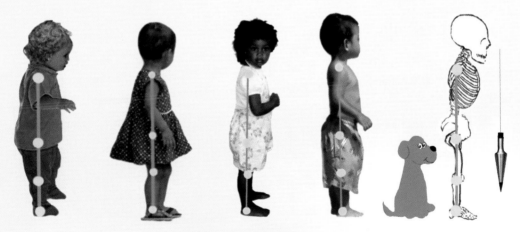

When babies learn how to balance upright, the weight-bearing joints—ankles, knees, hips and shoulders (yellow dots above)—are are precisely stacked up, one one on top of the other, along the vertical axis of gravity or "plumb line". This is true of every healthy child in the world who is born with the normally functioning "working parts".

9

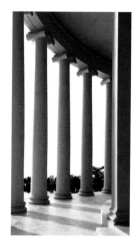

Stone columns or pillars have been used for centuries to hold up temples and other buildings. Some of them are still standing after thousands of years. This is possible because they distribute the forces of gravity directly through the vertical axis.

Although the bones of our legs are not perfectly straight (the *femur*, or thigh bone, has a pronounced curve) they are designed to work in relation to the foot bones and the pelvis in order to distribute the weight of the head, torso and forces of gravity, directly through the **vertical axis of gravity**. As long as the feet are properly aligned to support the leg bones, and the pelvis is positioned to bring each weight-bearing joint along the center line, the legs are able to provide the same solid support that pillars do.

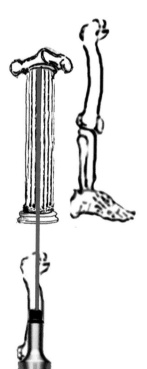

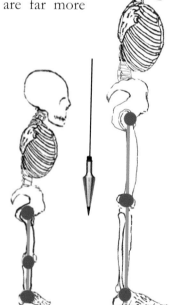

Of course, human legs are far more complex than stone columns. For one thing, our bones are alive, just as we are. They articulate or meet each other at joints that bend. One such joint is the knee, which makes it possible for us to bend our legs and move through space.

All natural movement requires a particular relationship between aligned bones and elastic muscles that support healthy joints and conform to the fundamental human design. This design provides for movement that is not only solid and aligned, but also fluid and serves to provide a shock absorbing feature.

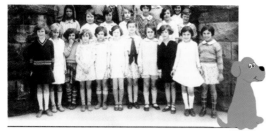

Standing Then ...

Not many years ago, most American children enjoyed the support of aligned leg bones, whether they were standing on both legs or only one (below). This allowed for the forces of gravity to be distributed along the central axis.

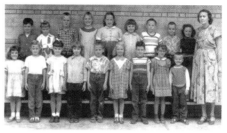

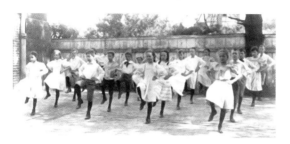

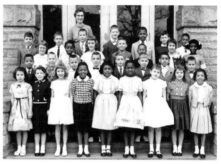

... and Now

It is rare today for school-age children to still have the support of solid, aligned leg bones.

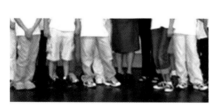

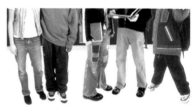

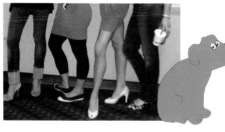

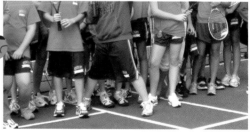

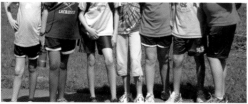

Without the support of aligned legs, the forces of gravity begin to bear down onto joints and intervertebral discs, and, over the ensuing years, a multitude of chronic structural problems develop.

Children who never lose their original natural alignment exhibit remarkable natural strength. Many participate in village and family life by carrying water on their heads and siblings on their backs—and do these things with ease. We think of this as "back-breaking" work, yet when aligned bones carry the load, even children can do this with very little effort.

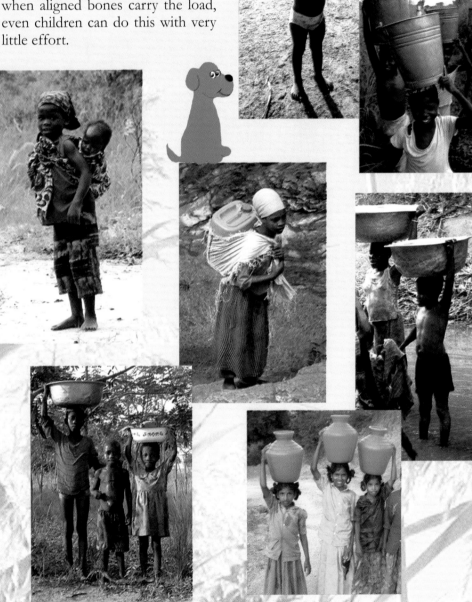

What *Real, Effortless* Fitness Looks Like

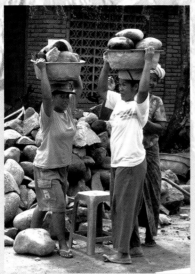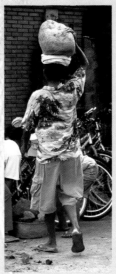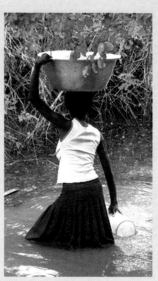

Adults who carry heavy loads on their heads with ease are not strong because they do this, they are able to successfully carry such heavy loads because their bones are aligned. This is the hallmark of being naturally strong.

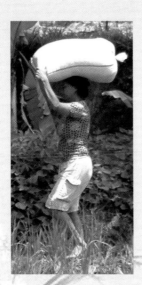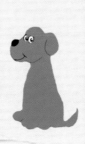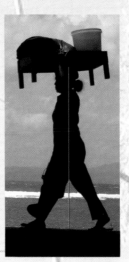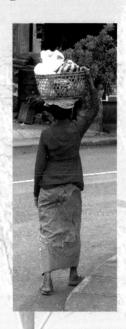

Some women carry heavy loads on their heads day in and day out for decades without ever developing pain or spinal problems. Such women might have never have heard of a "gym" or yoga, yet they are characterized by natural flexibility, authentic strength and a lack of struggle.

Partners with Gravity

Because these people's weight-bearing joints are aligned along the vertical axis, their spines are able to remain fully open, free of any compression. The lengthened, rising spine supports the head from below, allowing the neck to be long and relaxed. A minimum of muscle tension is required for these people to perform daily activities. Because of this, no matter what they are doing, they are able to feel comfortably relaxed.

These are the conditions that not only maintain flexibility, but preserve authentic strength and enduring vitality into old age. Such is the evolutionary design of our species, no matter where in the world we happen to be born. While all healthy children discover the central axis (without knowing, of course, that they have done this), few adults in technologically advanced places maintain this alignment past early childhood. While the incidence of those who report back pain at some point—not to mention a host of other structurally related disorders—tops 80% in the modern world, this figure drops dramatically in those places where people live with few modern "conveniences", such as cars, washing machines, computers, lawn mowers, power tools and "easy chairs", all of which contribute to a more sedentary lifestyle.

However, it is important to consider that it is less about one's level of activity than *how* the activity is performed that makes the difference. This explains why so many people injure themselves while exercising and physically exerting themselves.

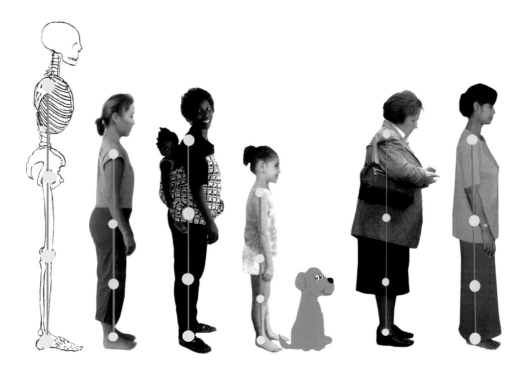

Victims of Gravity

Pulling joints off the vertical axis has a collapsing effect. Gravitational forces are unable to be distributed through a vertical line, and the weight of the head bears down (like a pile of rocks!) on the spine and joints throughout the body.

Over time, joints weaken and are easily strained and injured. The spine is under constant assault and unable to support itself. Straining muscles must pick up the slack, contributing to a long list of aches and pains. Ligaments and cartilage wear out over decades of misuse and give way to "wear-and-tear" conditions such as osteoarthritis. Constant compression of the spine provokes other conditions, such as muscles spasms, herniated discs, pinched nerves, spinal stenosis, and "degenerative disc disease". Hip and knee replacement surgeries are common in people who have lost structural support, since constant strain is put on the weight-bearing joints in movements as simple as bending over or getting in and out of a chair. Needless to say, such people are prone to injury.

Fatigue is a common symptom in people with a collapsed structure, along with general stiffness and vague and nagging aches and pains. The nervous system is under constant assault, and loss of physical vitality becomes a self-perpetuating vicious cycle with each problem being compounded and multiplied. The good news is that people of any age can learn to align their bones and find relief from many of these problems. It doesn't happen without practice, but it does work!

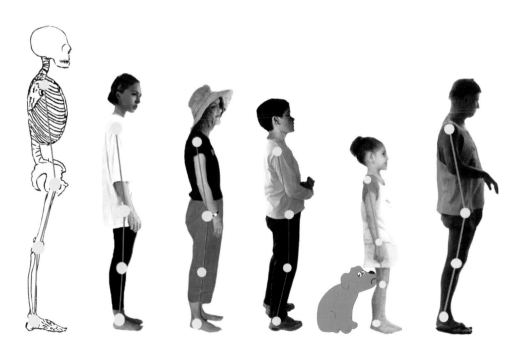

Fighting Against Gravity

In an attempt to counteract the collapse that occurs when bones are not aligned, we have adopted a society-wide misperception of what "good posture" is and how it is supposed to look. Typical instructions for implementing this stance include tucking the butt, sucking in the belly, lifting the chest and pulling the shoulders back. Many people who stand like this are also in the habit of locking or hyper-extending their knees.

This "ideal" posture that dominates our current "fitness" paradigm, compresses the spine and requires a large amount of muscular tension to hold the body "up". Because building strength in muscles often comes with the benefit of increased stamina, and stretching often brings temporary relief from tension, it can sometimes take a while for accumulating problems to appear. For this reason, people who inhabit this stance will sometimes become "addicted" to their exercise routines, needing them in order to feel good. Sometimes it is not until people pass through their middle years that they begin to notice the back pain that develops whenever they go for a hike, the stiffness that greets them in the morning, the bunions developing on their feet, and the knee or hip that hurts after a yoga class. *Any exercise that is done with a misaligned skeleton reinforces habits of mechanical use that are the cause of the problem in the first place.* It can be disappointing to discover that many of our efforts have been leading in the wrong direction. However, the good news is, that with determined practice, one can learn to exercise in ways that gradually return the body to its natural "home base".

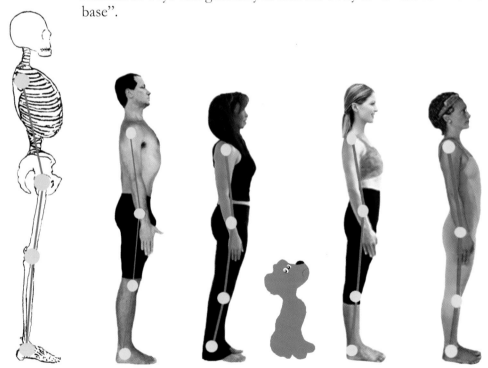

Have you ever seen a baby or toddler
standing with her chest lifted up?
Not likely!

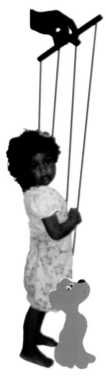

It is strange to imagine a very young
child standing in such an unnatural way,
even though this is a characteristic stance
for many adults today. This is what
would happen if puppet strings were
attached at the front side of this child's
body, pulling it forward and up, off the
axis. The real problem with this is that it
takes the weight-bearing joints off the
center line, tucking the pelvis and
arching (i.e., compressing) the spine.
This resembles the stance of the people
on the facing page.

Cut the strings and down she goes …

Without the "tension" of puppet
strings to hold her up, she
collapses. *Misalignment of bones off
of the central axis is the primary cause
of slouching, a fact that is widely
overlooked.*

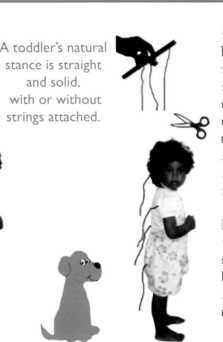

A toddler's natural
stance is straight
and solid,
with or without
strings attached.

f puppet strings attached at
he back of this toddler were
ut, she would not collapse.
nstead, she would continue to
e supported by an interplay
f *aligned* bones and *elastic*
nuscles that are both relaxed
nd engaged. Healthy muscles
re neither chronically
ontracted nor slack.

This clearly demonstrates the
tability provided by aligned
ones when a child discovers
he central axis of gravity that
llows easy balance in an
ipright position.

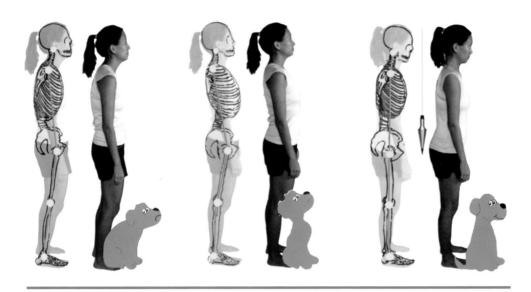

Aligned, "Happy Dog" Puppets

A "Happy Dog" puppet stands *as if* imaginary puppet strings were attached at strategic points along the back of the body. Of course,

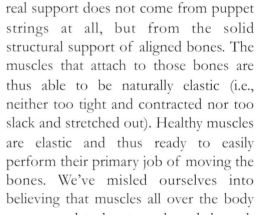

real support does not come from puppet strings at all, but from the solid structural support of aligned bones. The muscles that attach to those bones are thus able to be naturally elastic (i.e., neither too tight and contracted nor too slack and stretched out). Healthy muscles are elastic and thus ready to easily perform their primary job of moving the bones. We've misled ourselves into believing that muscles all over the body need to be strengthened through "working out".

This way of standing can look different to someone raised in a culture that teaches one to stand up straight by pulling the chest upward and pulling the shoulders back. (See facing page.)

Lifted Up, Tense Puppet

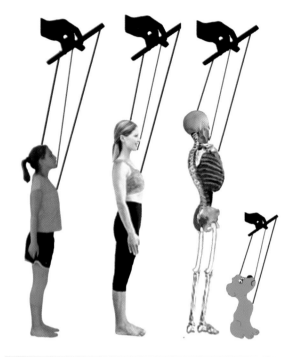

Imaginary puppet strings attached to the front of the body pull the body off the central axis. Deep tension is required to "hold" the body in this lifted-up stance, now that aligned bones are no longer available to do the job. As the chest and chin are pulled up, muscles along the spine tighten. It is ironic that many people practice *Tadasana* or Mountain Pose in yoga this way, a posture that is intended to invoke both solid groundedness and relaxation. Neither of these qualities is possible when gravity cannot be distributed through aligned bones and muscles are forced to work to maintain the misaligned position, rather than be able to relax.

Slouching, "Sad Dog" Puppet

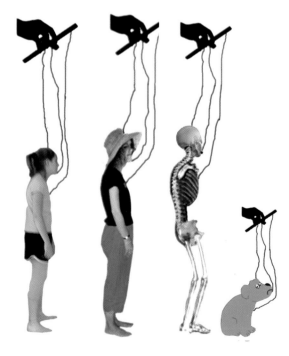

This is what would happen if you were standing in the "lifted-up" stance pictured above and the puppet strings were suddenly loosened. Without taut strings— i.e., without muscle tension— you would sink and collapse, since you would be unable to rely on aligned bones to support you. The models on the left are not that different from the ones above in that none of them is supported by aligned legs and an aligned pelvis. The ones above are simply using constant muscle tension to lift and hold themselves up in order to prevent the otherwise inevitable collapse. Much of the current emphasis on developing strength through gym workouts is an attempt to counteract chronic collapse.

Aligned Living = Comfortable Aging

People who age into their 70s, 80s and beyond, without ever losing natural alignment, enjoy extended spines, genuine strength, easy flexibility and enduring vitality. These are the benefits they reap from having lived their entire lives as "Happy Dogs".

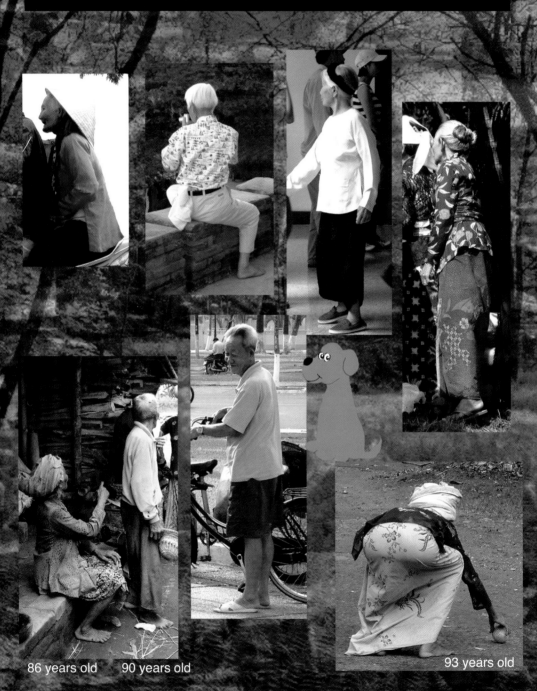

86 years old   90 years old   93 years old

Misaligned Living = Stiff and Painful Aging

This kind of collapse is considered to be an inevitable feature of aging, but is, actually, the result of decades of habitual "Sad Dog" posture. Each one of these people is characterized by a severely "tucked butt". At such time in the future that meaningful research is conducted that examines postural habits based on the actual human design, it will not be surprising if it is determined that structural misalignment plays a significant role in the development of such degenerative conditions as osteoarthritis and osteoporosis.

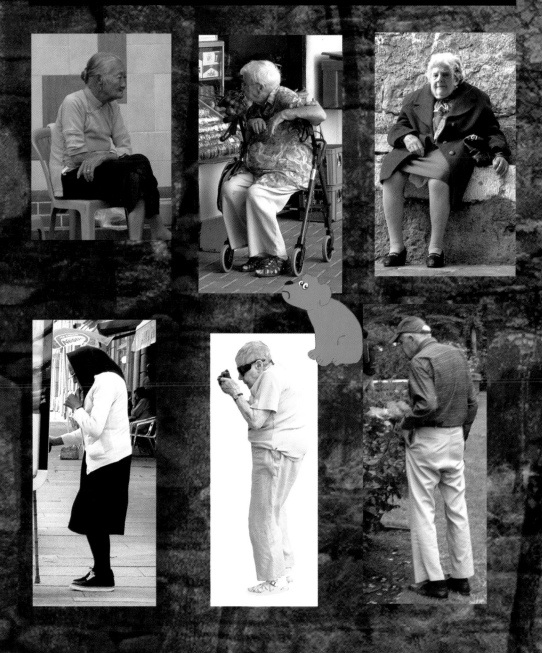

Working feet

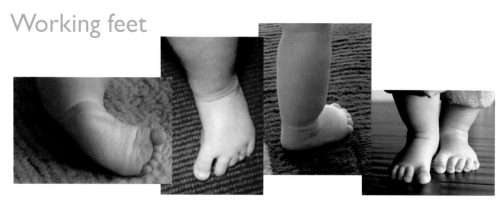

Healthy babies' feet are shaped like kidney beans (or croissants), with toes that grab the ground in order to aid balance. Babies often have a pad of fat that hides the primary medial arch, the actual height of which is revealed by the height of the top of the foot, above the arch. The lower leg bones, the *tibia* and *fibula*, form vertical lines that come to rest squarely on the ankle platform (*talus*), stabilized by ligaments that lash the ankle joint into place. The child's weight is distributed through the primary arch and out onto the heel, a thick bone that is well-designed for this purpose.

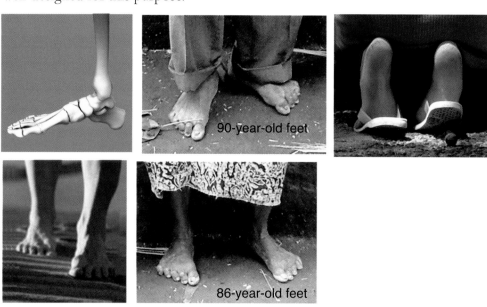

90-year-old feet

86-year-old feet

Adults who never lose what we all first knew as children are supported by feet that greatly resemble the architecture of children's feet. The body's weight is distributed more along the outside of the feet than we are accustomed to seeing in adults in the "modern world". The arches remain raised, the toes still grab the ground, and the ankle is aligned and stable. All of these features provide the ingredients for a lifetime of enduring structural support. Without the support of aligned foot bones, the integrity of the skeletal structure above begins to develop stresses that become compounded over the ensuing years.

Setting the stage for a lifetime of support

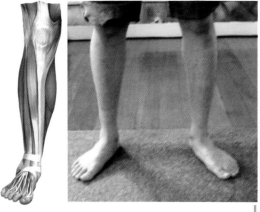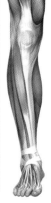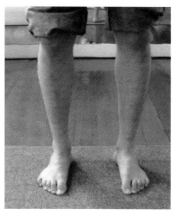

<table>
<tr><td>

Collapsed Feet
Weak Legs

</td><td>

Aligned Feet
Strong Legs

</td></tr>
</table>

This stance, with feet wide apart and ankles pronated (dropping inward), is very common today. The weight of the body is thrown onto the inside edges of the feet, causing the primary arches to flatten. This over-stretches the ligaments of the ankles that would otherwise hold the ankle in place. This also puts strain on the the knee and hip joints, that now lack structural support from below and are misshapen and distorted. This all adds up to a poor engineering design that cannot adequately support the structure above and will have far-reaching consequences in the years ahead.

Moments later, these same feet have been transformed. By learning to "tuck the heels" almost anyone can rearrange the bones of the feet to provide stable support. Once the heels are tucked, the arches are lifted, the toes are engaged and the ankles are no longer pronated or pushing off the ankle platform. While this is just a first step, one that will require persistent practice, it is essential to providing the support needed for a lifetime of solid strength that is free of tension and strain.

The arrangement of the bones of the feet determines whether the legs will function as solid foundational posts of support, or if, over time, they will undermine the stability of the skeleton above them.

Tuck your heels

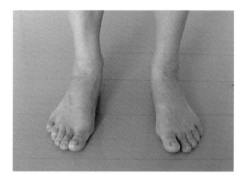

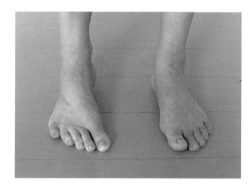

The following simple steps rearrange the bones and raise collapsing arches, stabilize pronated ankles and activate disengaged toes. Bunions often result from the weight of the body being thrust forward and pushed out through the joint of the big toes.

Step #1: Aim the toes of your right foot slightly toward the center. With the heel lifted only a fraction of an inch off the floor, hold onto the floor with your toes and the ball of your foot.

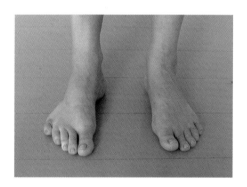

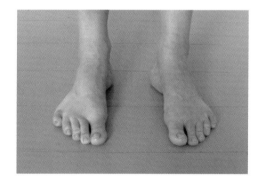

Step #2: Still holding on with the toes, turn your knee to the outside while "tucking" your heel under, bringing the outside edge of your heel onto the floor toward the center. Straighten your leg, square your hips, if necessary, and with equal weight on both legs, take a moment to experience the difference in how each leg feels.

Step #3: Repeat on the left side. Sense how this leg feels now. While this is not a quick fix and must be repeated many times, along with other exercises (Chapter 5) until the muscles that support aligned feet are reconfigured, your feet will gradually re-shape. You should now be able to see your heels in a mirror, along with lifted arches and engaged toes.

Before and After Tucking the Heels

Side A shows the leg before the heel is tucked. Here we see a collapsed arch, pronated ankle, disengaged toes and an unsupported, inwardly turned knee. Distorted muscles—some overly contracted, others overly stretched—are clearly visible through the length of the leg. This arrangement of bones also changes the way the head of the thigh bone (*femur*) sits in the hip socket, putting great stress on the ligaments and contributing to destruction of cartilage in the joint. This situation often results, decades later, in hip and/or knee replacement surgery. The leg muscles are working in an unbalanced way, visible through tension in the calf muscles.

Side B shows the leg after the heel is tucked. The weight now lands on the outside of the foot and heel, the arch is raised, the toes are active in providing support and balance, and the ankle is now supported on top of the ankle platform (*talus*). The other joints of the leg, the knee and hip, are also both aligned and supported by properly configured muscles, tendons and ligaments. The muscles of the leg are balanced front to back and side to side, so that no muscles are overly contracted or overly stretched. People who never lose the support of aligned legs are much less likely to be candidates for hip or knee replacement, as well as back pain, neck pain and a long list of complaints common to people whose feet do not provide adequate support.

The importance of aligned foot bones is largely overlooked in terms of the key role they play in support for the whole body. Misaligned foot bones are usually the cause of a long list of foot problems, from bunions to plantar fasciitis. Learning how to align the feet can also lead to resolving chronic back and hip pain.

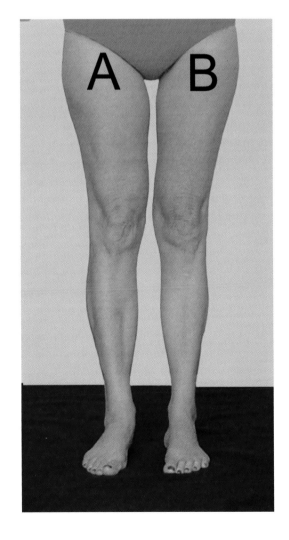

The Role of Mindfulness

Mindfulness is a quality of attention that is directed, without analysis or judgement, to one's experience in present time. By focusing your awareness on whatever you happen to be seeing, hearing, touching, smelling, tasting—as well as sensations and "feelings" you may notice, you stay anchored right here, right now, in the reality of this moment. Rather than being swept away or "lost" in thoughts of the past or the future, you are here, right now with what actually is, not what is imagined. A growing body of evidence points to the fact that cultivating mindfulness can improve one's overall quality of life.

A willingness to be mindful is a necessary ingredient for putting principles of natural alignment into practice. This is far from easy for anyone, but the benefits are unending. Focusing your attention on the alignment of your bones serves as a useful and concrete tool for developing greater awareness. Presence is not just a state of mind but a state of body/mind. As you practice turning inward to a "center of being" that is as physically deep as the marrow of your bones, you develop a capacity for meditating on the body all day long. Paying attention to how you sit at the computer, bend to tie your shoes, practice yoga, lift a child into your arms or jog around the block, works to develop a gradually deepening capacity for being fully present with yourself.

Mindfulness tends to be contagious. When we behave mindlessly, dashing around in a frantic swirl of busyness, we teach our children to be this way, too. When we model a calm, centered demeanor, even in the throes of our ordinarily busy lives, we bequeath these qualities to our children, who are the beneficiaries of our own enhanced state of peace and equanimity. In time, mindfulness contributes to a greater sense of our own happiness. Our own happiness is one of the greatest gifts we can give to our children, who are profoundly affected by the underlying condition of a parent's mind.

Today's children are growing up in an environment of almost constant stimulation, with fewer and fewer opportunities for them to interact with Nature. This can keep them cut off from experiencing their connection to the natural world, as well as knowing themselves to be an inseparable part of that world.

Too often, adults, while confusing sensuality with sexuality, send indirect signals to children to shut down actually *feeling* the sensations that come with having a body and being alive. Giving acceptance to a child as a fully human physical "creature" with a discernible "felt" life inside the skin, bestows acceptance of oneself as a valuable participant in a great and wondrous world. Such understanding sows the seeds of acceptance of others, as well, and nurtures a deep caring for the world of which we are all a part.

Such is the nature of mindfulness. Aligned bones promote and support mindfulness.

A Few Words About Breathing

The diaphragm is the primary muscle of respiration. When breathing is natural, it takes on the shape of an open parachute on each exhalation and flattens down somewhat on each inhalation. Attached to the inside of the rib cage, the diaphragm depends on the rib cage being aligned properly in order to be able to function efficiently. A collapsed chest, or one that is over-lifted, distorts fibers of the diaphragm, impairing its ability to move with easy elasticity.

Babies demonstrate effortless, gentle breathing that is unrestrained by any unnecessary muscle tension. Except when they are in distress, babies and toddlers breathe with an easy rising and falling away of each breath. Watch a baby breathe, and the breath seems to touch everywhere in the torso. Put your hand on a baby's back or the sides of the rib cage, and you will be able to feel the touch of the breath under your hand.

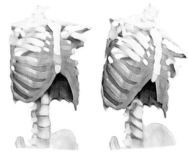

Aligned rib cage
& diaphragm

Distorted
rib cage

Breathing and relaxation are inseparable, with each affecting the other: Anxiety creates breath-holding and breath-holding creates anxiety. By the same token, "taking a deep breath" is often misunderstood to mean sucking in as much air as possible into the chest. Natural breathing creates a whisper-soft fullness throughout the widest, bottom-most part of the lungs and can be felt throughout the back. Fast, hard breathing occurs naturally when we run or exert ourselves, but, when we are at rest, breathing happens softly and quietly on its own, without any manipulation.

This can be easier said than done, particularly for anyone with longstanding patterns of restricted breathing and entrenched muscular tension. It helps to carve out time on a regular basis to first align your bones and then focus the mind on observing and experiencing the subtle sensations of each breath.

You may have difficulty knowing how to let go, unconsciously sensing that you could fall apart if you don't remain "on guard" by holding yourself together with tension. It can come as a huge relief to discover that aligned bones provide the structural safety that supports us when we finally learn how to let go. Think of yourself as having an inner and an outer body. The inner body is all the bones, the outer body is everything else. With the inner body in place, the outer body can relax. Bring your attention to your breath often. As you inhale, visualize the breath moving up the full length of your back. This encourages the diaphragm to work in a natural way. As you exhale, sense the breath moving down the front of your spine, causing the floor of the pelvis to widen and the sit bones to move apart, as your "outer body" melts away and lets go of all tension.

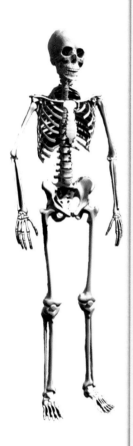

TWO

The Skeleton

The skeleton is the framework of support for all the body's systems, including those that regulate breathing, circulation of blood, digestion of food and the basic functions of the nervous system. Besides producing blood cells and storing minerals, the bones provide the body's form and underlying structure.

Much like the support posts found inside the walls of a house, skeletal bones provide the structure for the efficient arrangement of internal "plumbing" and "electrical wiring". Like the posts in a house, they must conform to the laws of gravity and verticality.

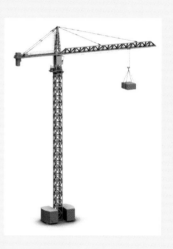

The musculoskeletal system works much like the design of a building crane; both are systems of pulleys and levers that employ "correct" tension of the pulleys (muscles) to move the levers (bones). It is not difficult to imagine how unstable the workings of the upper part of a crane would be if the alignment of the foundation were skewed. The balanced relationship between pulleys and levers would be thrown off, creating imbalance and tension (i.e., muscle tension), as often happens with the human body.

The essential role of the skeleton's natural alignment may be the single most overlooked and misunderstood factor relating to overall health and well being today. No one would question the importance of a healthy diet, appropriate exercise and the reduction of unnecessary stress to overall good health. However, the importance of aligned bones to an integrated whole that provides support for healthy functioning of all the body's systems has been, until now, largely overlooked.

The Musculoskeletal System

The primary job of muscles is to move bones. This makes it possible for us to sit, stand, bend, walk, and engage in all other types of movement.

While muscles do play a secondary role in providing support to the skeleton, it is a serious mistake to think of muscles as being in charge of holding us up or holding us together. This notion can lead to chronic, unnecessary tension and robs the bones of their important role. Misalignment of bones is the cause of much of the muscular pain and discomfort experienced by millions of people today.

Misaligned bones force the muscles that are attached to them to be either overly shortened or overly lengthened. This situation has given rise to the current popularity of stretching exercises and muscle strengthening techniques, a recent phenomenon in the several hundred-thousand years of human existence. Normally, in the course of everyday activities, the body's natural interplay between *aligned* bones and *elastic* muscles, keeps the muscles naturally toned and the joints open and flexible.

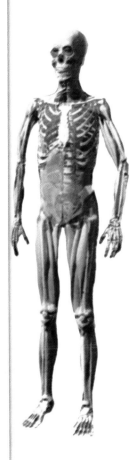

Creating imbalance in the musculoskeletal system through unnaturally developed "strength" restricts the range of motion of joints and compresses the spine. Such artificial strength is only temporary and requires continuous repetition of exercises to be maintained. The same is true with flexibility, a quality that is either a natural by-product of an aligned body or something that must be maintained through regular stretching exercises. Any improvement one gets often fade once the exercises are stopped.

Certain kinds of exercise may bring temporary relief from stored up muscular tension and pain; however, this release is only a short-term remedy if alignment issues are not addressed. Exercising with misaligned bones can further entrench habits that perpetuate the return of tension and stiffness, which is then temporarily relieved by more exercise, and, thus, a vicious cycle is set in place that undermines both authentic strength and natural flexibility.

The Respiratory System

Breathing is essential to life. Every cell in the body requires oxygen to function and thrive.

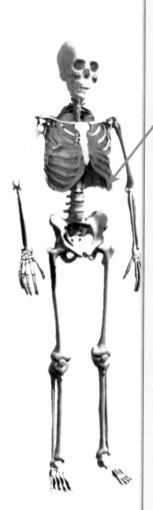

The diaphragm is the primary muscle of respiration. A dome-shaped muscle that separates the chest cavity from the abdominal cavity, the diaphragm draws oxygen into the lungs by contracting and flattening down and then pushing disposable carbon dioxide out of the body by relaxing back up into its parachute-like shape.

A rib cage that is either collapsed or lifted-up with tension distorts the muscle fibers of the diaphragm, impinging on its ability to remain elastic and perform its important task in an efficient way. Countless techniques are taught, both modern and ancient, as ways to manipulate the breath for various purposes, most especially relaxation. *Surprisingly, the importance of skeletal alignment for supporting natural breathing is still virtually unrecognized.*

Breathing intimately affects the autonomic nervous system, which comprises the sympathetic (fight or flight) and parasympathetic (relaxation) aspects of the nervous system. Breathing like a baby, softly, gently and naturally, is the most effective way to promote relaxation.

Breathing interrelates with other bodily systems, as well, such as supplying the oxygen that is delivered by the circulatory system and which serves as food for all the body's cells.

The human organism can survive for many years with less than efficient breathing. Yet consequences of restricted breathing accumulate over the course of many years, affecting the function of all the systems and degrading overall health and wellbeing.

The Circulatory System

The circulatory system is responsible for managing the flow of blood and distribution of oxygen and nutrients throughout the body.

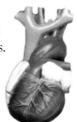

Veins and arteries are like miniature garden hoses that function best as open channels. Chronic narrowing or crimping of these channels diminishes the flow of blood and thus the amount of oxygen that is available to each of the billions of cells of the body.

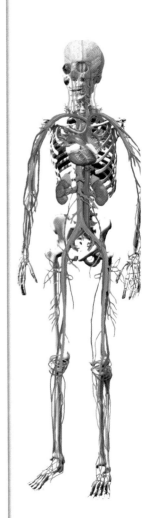

A chest that is chronically collapsed compresses the heart, which is a three-dimensional organ with valves and "tubes". Collapse of the chest cavity distorts the natural arrangement of these various heart components. *Considering the epidemic of heart conditions plaguing so many people, the misalignment of the heart itself (along with its maze of blood vessels) may be a seriously overlooked factor in addressing heart disease.* Indeed, rarely does a health professional discuss whether there is adequate spaciousness in all directions to support a non-compressed, well-functioning heart. If the heart were an important part in a car's engine, such misalignment would be considered to be a serious problem.

Collapse of the chest, however, is not the only problem. An over-corrected stance that lifts the ribcage and holds it up with muscular tension puts a different type of stress on the circulatory system. Muscular tension creates pressure against the walls of blood vessels, narrowing the internal channels and impeding the optimal "relaxed" flow of blood.

Once again, we see the importance of an aligned skeleton for providing necessary support for the open and efficient functioning of the an essential body system.

Vital Organs & Digestive System

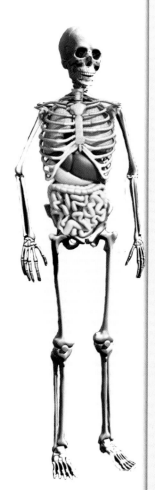

Neatly packaged within the torso is a complex arrangement of many organs—heart, lungs, kidneys, liver, stomach, pancreas, gall bladder, small intestine, large intestine—and all the multiple tubes and valves that connect them with each other.

Living up to their name, these organs are vital to the life and overall health of the body and share a well-filled, limited space in the torso. If these organs, which are connected to each other and other body parts by various tubes and valves, are compressed and pushed together by chronic structural collapse, their efficient function is impaired. It seems obvious that this would have both immediate and long-term effects on one's health.

One hopes that research will begin to consider the relationship between structural integrity and the functioning of vital organs when examining the causes and contributing factors that may play a part in the current epidemic of certain digestive disorders and a number of modern "lifestyle" diseases. A healthy diet, which has been determined to be essential to good health, is supported by a complex digestive process that includes the release of digestive juices and enzymes and the absorption and assimilation of nutrients, along with the elimination of waste products. Any disruption along the prescribed physical path that food takes from "in" to "out", is likely to take a toll over the decades of one's life.

While the human body is more complex and adaptable than an automobile, this analogy is valid in that alignment of such parts as valves, pistons and timing belts is essential to the smooth operation of the car. Likewise, organs of digestion, elimination and detoxification rely on correct alignment of the skeletal structure that supports them, and any impairment of their functions can have serious consequences.

The Nervous System

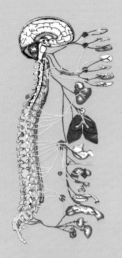

The nervous system is the most complex of all the body's mechanisms, coordinating and controlling actions of all the other systems and organs, receiving, processing and transmitting messages back and forth from the brain and interpreting information from the external environment.

The spinal cord is the primary neural pathway connecting the brain and peripheral nervous system, which encompasses all the body's parts and functions. This bundle of nerve tissue and cells is encased within the vertebral canal, protected by the bony structure of the spine.

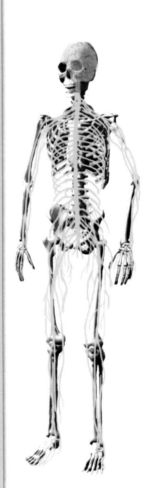

Disruption of natural alignment of the spine can lead to pressure on nerves that often results in pain, numbness and a long list of medically recognized musculoskeletal conditions. Beyond contributing to general pain and dysfunction of the central nervous system, skeletal misalignment may also play a far greater role in contributing to other health conditions than has been previously understood. The spinal cord's ability to serve as an open conduit that governs the functions of the peripheral nervous system and its various parts—the somatic (movement), enteric (digestive) and autonomic systems (stress/relaxation)—may play a significant role in otherwise misunderstood conditions such as fibromyalgia and chronic fatigue syndrome, to name only the most obvious.

Alignment of the skeleton also affects the respiratory system, closely related to the sympathetic (fight or flight) aspect of the autonomic nervous system and the parasympathetic (relaxation response) aspect. In this way, the state of one's "carriage" not only affects the quality of breathing, but one's state of mind, as well.

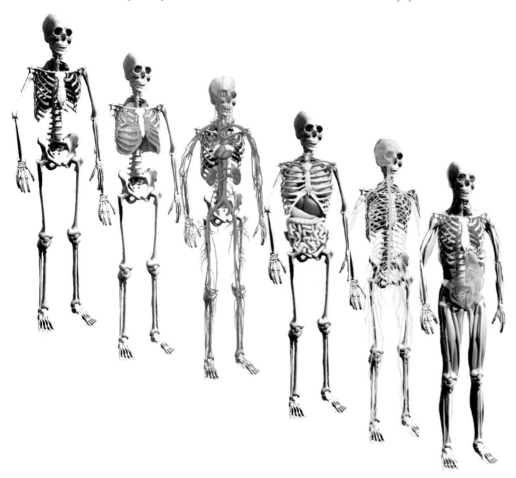

Picturing the human body as a 3-D puzzle of many intricate,
interrelated parts helps to make clear the importance of having each "piece" of
that puzzle—blood vessel, internal organ, muscle, or nerve—in its rightful
place. With the support of an aligned skeleton, these essential pieces are able to
function together with efficiency and provide the necessary conditions that are
the cornerstone of good health and comfortable living.

To date, there appears to be no research whatsoever that examines the overall
health of people who maintain qualities of "naturalness", such as toddlers and
a select, yet rapidly diminishing, group of adults in the world. Once such
research finally gets underway, countless doors of insight will open that will
broaden our understanding of the essential role played by aligned bones in
supporting good health and wellbeing. The recognition of the key role played
by the body's underlying framework may well represent the next big
breakthrough in "modern medicine".

"A place for everything, and everything in its place."

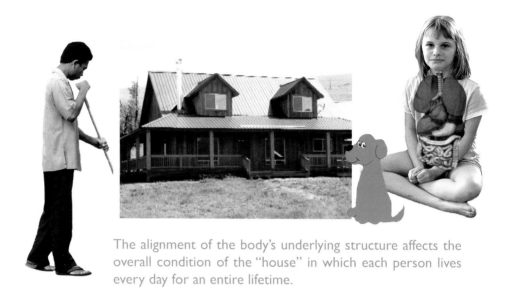

The alignment of the body's underlying structure affects the overall condition of the "house" in which each person lives every day for an entire lifetime.

The fact that so many children spend hours every day in a state of collapse while sitting in front of computer and television screens or slumped over their desks in school, presents a serious and growing health problem. Even when they are aware of the problem, most parents, teachers and health professionals are at a loss to know how to address it.

In fact, fewer and fewer adults today know how to inhabit their own bodies in healthy ways and are, thus, unable to serve as role models of good alignment for children.

Ignoring the relationship between aligned bones and one's health is not much different than expecting the plumbing and wiring of a house to work well when the house itself is falling down.

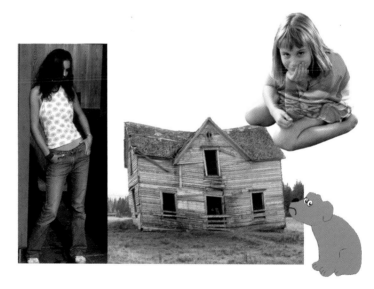

Three   Keeping Children Naturally Aligned
Habit patterns are established early.

Don't train your child to be a "Sad Dog!"

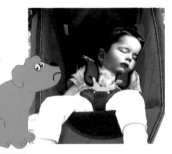

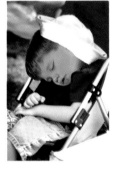

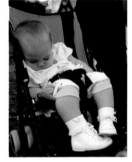

Many strollers and sitting devices in use today promote tucking of the tailbone and collapsing of the spine. Some children spend many hours a week buckled into positions that train muscles along the front of the torso and hip flexor muscles to be habitually contracted. This sets up patterns that will help define how a child sits and moves throughout his or her lifetime.

Babies everywhere begin to lengthen the spine from the moment they are born, leaving the curled up fetal position behind once they are no longer a fetus.

Protect the integrity of your child's spine

Certain strollers can be modified by placing a child-sized wedge* or folded cloth under the sit bones to raise the back edge of the pelvis and place it into a "Happy Dog" position. A good rule of thumb would be to create whatever conditions support optimal length of your child's spine.

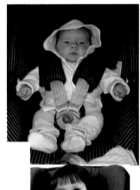

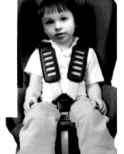

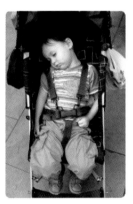

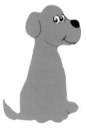

* See Appendix

36

Give your child every opportunity
to remain a natural "Happy Dog!"

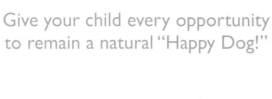

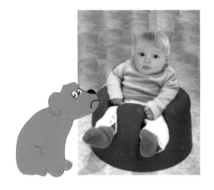

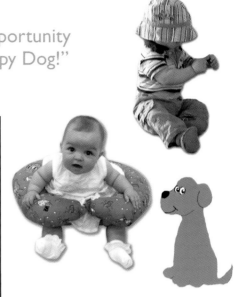

It may be a mistake to use sitting devices such as the one pictured here before a child is able to sit upright on his or her own. Any sitting surface that dips lower at the back tucks the pelvis, throws the weight of the spine off the sacral platform, shortens muscles in the front of the body and collapses the spine.

Let your child learn to sit up naturally, with a fully extended spine. Placing stabilizing support *around* a child that allows her to find her sit bones is a better alternative to certain kinds of sitting devices. Even so, it's helpful to remember that, throughout the ages, babies everywhere have simply learned how sit up on their own through a process of trial and error.

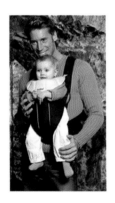 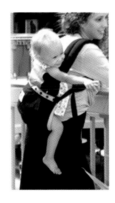 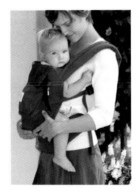 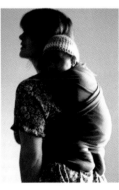

In addition to providing physical and emotional closeness that a young child enjoys when "worn" by a parent, a variety of baby carriers place the child's pelvis in the position that supports a fully lengthened spine. Avoid carriers that keep the child's spine in a "slumped" position. Such carriers can pose a danger to an infant if the air passage is cut off and can promote "tucking" after the first few months of life.

More things to do as a parent

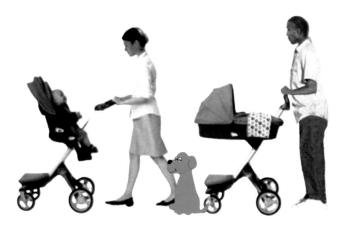

There are scores of models of baby equipment from which to choose today. Compare what is available and, when possible, purchase devices that best support your child's natural alignment through each developmental stage. Stay away from products with "bucket" style seating that causes the pelvis to tuck under or those that can't be easily adapted or modified.

If your child's stroller causes "tucking" of the pelvis, put a baby-size wedge-shaped cushion* under the sit bones to place the pelvis in the "Happy Dog" position.

See Appendix for how to order a "Baby Wedgie™".

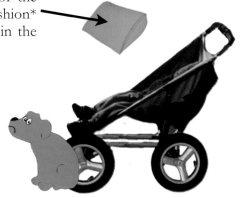

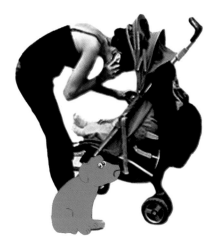

Who knows how early babies imprint what they see in those around them? Babies may be far more keen observers than we have previously understood.

Be a good role model for your baby. Learn how to put principles of natural alignment into practice in your own daily life (See Part Two) while sitting, standing, walking and bending, as well as lifting and carrying your baby.

* See Appendix

38

As babies become "kids"

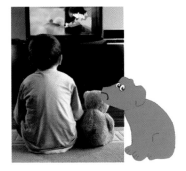 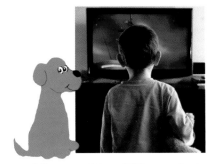

Monitor how your children are sitting while watching TV or playing video games. In the same way that you would not give your child a sugary snack in place of a nutritious meal, there is nothing wrong with establishing a rule that says that in order to be able to watch television or use the computer, these activities must be done as "Happy Dogs". You can provide a small wedge-shaped cushion that makes sitting upright easier.

The child pictured at left is not yet two years old. Like so many children today, he is already beginning to "tuck the butt" when he sits on a flat surface. Notice the rounding in the lower back and the shortening in his neck. He uses his hand on the floor to help support himself, but when he has a lift under his sit bones, his body remembers how to support itself.

Pay attention to how your child is wearing a backpack. Backpacks should be worn high on the back and not be excessively heavy.

Having information to share with your children, such as the images in this book, can be very useful in helping them understand why you are concerned about the way they sit at the computer, carry a backpack or play sports.

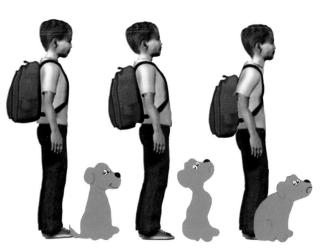

This little boy is doing a good job of sitting in "Happy Dog" mode, in spite of the poor design of his chair. By sitting on the edge of the chair, he is able to widen his sit bones out behind him and

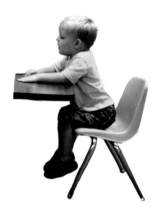

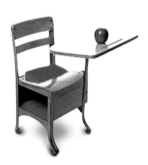

maintain the length of his spine. He would be better served to be sitting on a chair with a forward-tilted seat or a wedge cushion to help "park" his pelvis. The desk surface is too high for him, causing his shoulders to lift up around his ears. Desktops that incline and are adjustable are ideal.

Unfortunately, most school desk chairs dip lower at the back of the seat, forcing the pelvis into a backward tilt. Talk with your school administrators about replacing such desks and chairs with ones that are more appropriate. Students benefit greatly when they are provided with ways to sit that help place the pelvis in "Happy Dog" mode. If your school cannot afford to do this, you can hold an informational event for parents and initiate a fund-raising drive for the purchase of simple sitting wedges or large balls, both of which provide students with many benefits (See Appendix).

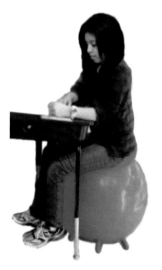

Introduce concepts of natural alignment to your students. Include details from Part Two "Guidelines and Instructions" as part of the daily curriculum, reminding your students periodically throughout the day to bring their attention to how they are sitting or standing. Help them remember to be "Happy Dogs". Not only will your students learn how to be supported by an aligned skeleton in everything they do, they also will be increasing the flow of oxygenated blood to their brains, essential to learning. Another important benefit is that you will be helping them to cultivate their capacity for mindfulness, a quality that will serve them well throughout their lives.

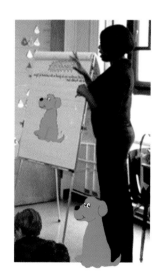

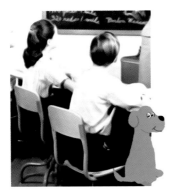

Encourage your students to not rely on backrests. This helps them keep the sit bones wide and promotes length of the spine as they lean forward from the hips toward the desktop. They can also be taught how to use a backrest in a helpful way (See Part Two).

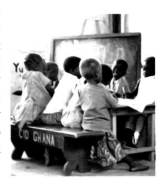

Remind them when you see some "Sad Dogs" in the room. This will help them remember that repositioning the pelvis when sitting is the first step in building a foundation for structural support.

Teach by example. By inhabiting your own body in a way that is aligned and relaxed, you will be planting seeds of self-awareness in your students. Over time, these seeds will begin to sprout and then grow. In the years ahead, they will bear fruit as the children mature and embody the important lessons you have taught them.

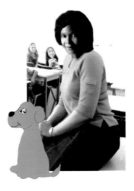

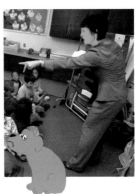

When teaching physical education or coaching sports

Inform children about how to move with sit bones behind them, fully-lengthened spines and knees that track to the outside. Model this for them

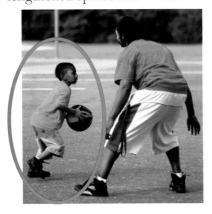

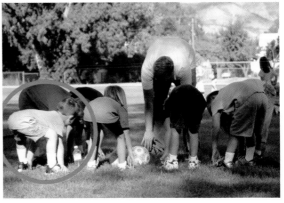

Three million children suffer from sports-related injuries each year, while millions more suffer from chronic "unexplained" pain. It is the two children, circled above in red, rather than the adults, who are modeling healthy habits of movement and have lengthened, open spines.

Naturally aligned children move with ease,
while maintaining extended spines and open joints.

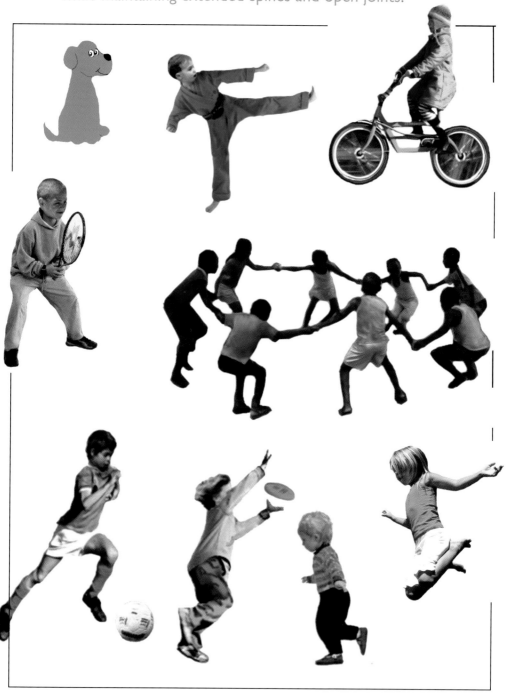

Exercise offers many benefits, but *how* we exercise determines whether
or not we reinforce habits that support good health
over the long run.

Children with compromised spines and restricted joints
move with effort and strain.

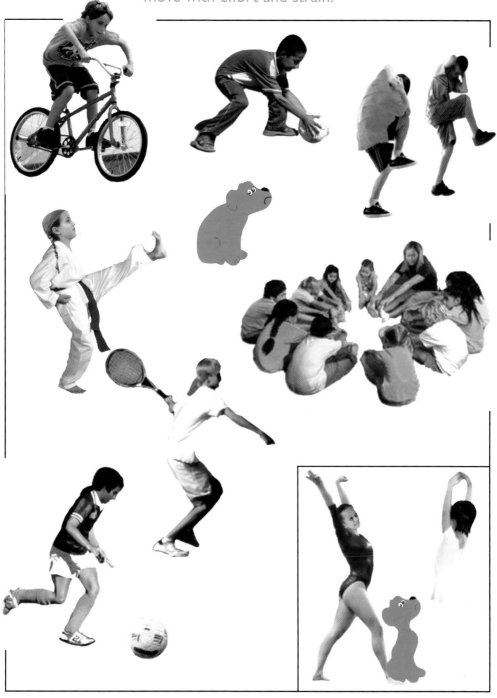

Exercising with misaligned bones not only entrenches poor habits of
use in the body, it often results in strain and injury.

The spine as the conduit for neural impulses.

A misaligned spine interferes with the ability to fully relax.

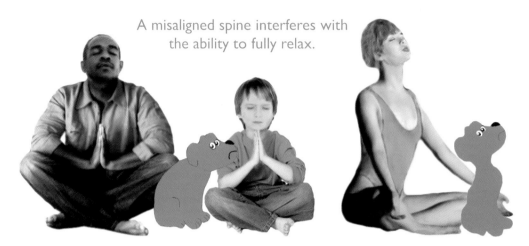

A growing body of evidence indicates that meditation offers many benefits that promote mental, emotional and physical health. One of these benefits is the cultivation of self-awareness, a key component to being more relaxed. Misaligned bones interfere with muscles being able to fully relax. Because meditation and relaxation techniques help stabilize the nervous system, these practices are successfully being introduced as ways to support children who struggle with learning disabilities and conditions such as ADHD.

An aligned spine promotes relaxation.

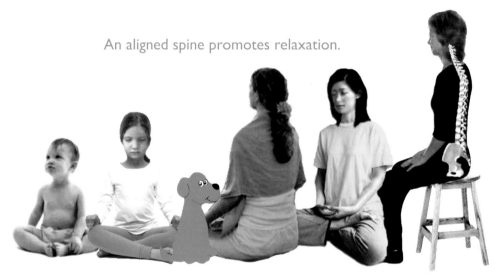

Very young children sit quite naturally in a perfect meditation posture, supported on an aligned pelvis with a self-supporting, lengthened spine. This promotes relaxed muscles and a calm state of mind. Energy is able to move freely through the body, unobstructed by the misalignment and tension as seen at the top of this page. Only with the support of aligned bones are muscles able to fully relax, making a deep state of relaxation possible.

What does it mean to be strong?

Who is stronger?

*Is it a body builder
who can lift heavy weights with the strength of muscles on the surface of his body?*

*Or is it a small woman
who easily carries a heavy load of rocks on her head with the power and
"bone deep" strength of aligned bones?*

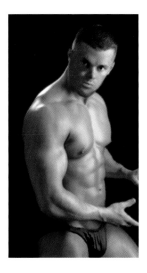

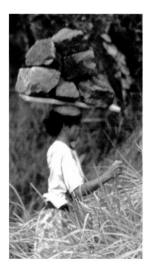

This type of strength

- Has its power in unnaturally developed muscles.

- Must be worked at repeatedly to be maintained.

- Compresses and shortens the spine.

- Limits the range of motion of many joints.

- Robs the diaphragm of natural elasticity.

- Stores chronic tension in bulky, overdeveloped muscles.

- Interferes with the parasympathetic nervous system (relaxation response).

This type of strength

- Has its power in an interplay of aligned bones and elastic muscles.

- Is reinforced in normal, everyday activities.

- Extends and opens the spine.

- Promotes freedom and flexibility of joints.

- Maintains natural elasticity of the diaphragm.

- Enhances elasticity of muscles.

- Tones the nervous system and promotes relaxation.

45

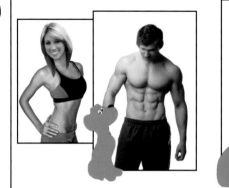

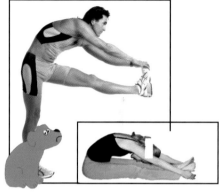

Artificially "sculpting" the body and developing specific muscles, such as "killer abs" and an overall "ripped" appearance, is a modern-day phenomenon. We have mistakenly convinced ourselves that muscle strength, not aligned bones, is required to hold us up. Not only does this concept go unquestioned, millions now believe that this culturally imposed standard is essential to health and happiness, neither of which, in the long run, is possible.

Exercise has many positive benefits which can include increased stamina, enhanced circulation, the burning of calories and fat, and temporary release of tension. Unfortunately, exercise that is done from a place of misalignment can also lead to injury and degenerative conditions of the joints and spine.

Can a distortion from what is natural be called "fitness" if it restricts natural movement of the diaphragm, stiffens joints, compresses the spine and turns muscles into over-developed storehouses of tension that never fully relax?

True fitness is effortless and relaxed and depends on flexible joints and an open spine.

Naturally aligned people are less likely to suffer injuries or be plagued by chronic aches and pains. They do not become "addicted" to exercise as a means to release pent up tension, as there is little tension stored in their muscles. They find physical activity to be both easy and enjoyable.

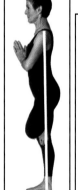

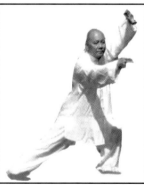

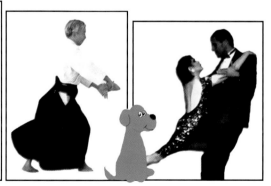

Experiencing the Body as a Forward-Turning Wheel

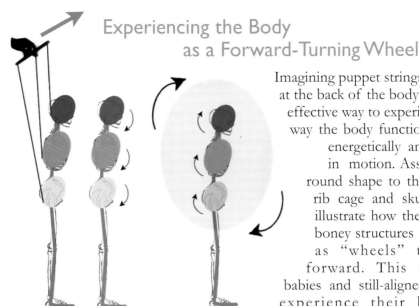

Imagining puppet strings attached at the back of the body is an effective way to experience the way the body functions both energetically and while in motion. Assigning a round shape to the pelvis, rib cage and skull helps illustrate how these three boney structures function as "wheels" turning forward. This is how babies and still-aligned adults experience their bodies, whether they are consciously aware of this fact or not. It is this upward and forward "pull" that most efficiently moves the body through space, in conformance with natural laws. Notice that the head is not pulled back, but drops slightly forward, leading the way.

In time, the smaller wheels can be experienced as one larger wheel continually rolling forward. This is the direction in which, if we are naturally aligned, we are "led" while walking, running, bending forward, getting up off the floor or out of a chair.

Such "forward-rolling" movement is always counter-balanced by a deep grounding connection into the earth, a connection that makes easeful movement possible in the first place. Think of a cat preparing to jump up onto a wall. The higher the wall, the more deeply the cat will crouch down, connecting itself more deeply into the earth as it draws up the "energy" it needs to leap forward and up. This energy is the "ground-reaction force" that appears to be integral to the design of all vertebrate species.

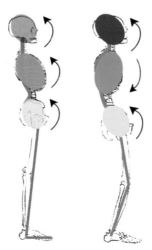

Turning any of the boney "wheels" in the wrong direction disrupts the body's ability to connect with this ground-reaction force. This leads to inefficient movement, tightness in muscles, stiffness in joints, compression in the spine, blockage of energy and the likelihood that even minor falls and accidents will result in injury and chronic pain problems. Veering off from the body's innate design around the central axis contributes to a host of problems that will only continue to grow in epidemic numbers until we, as modern-day humans, re-discover how our human bodies are designed to be inhabited for effortless, graceful movement.

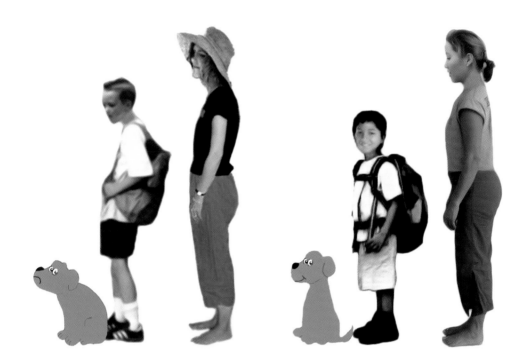

Children and adults can help each other remember to be mindful and pay attention to how each is sitting or standing. If you think of this as an adventure you are on together, with an aim toward each helping the other along the way, you are both more likely to be successful.

Returning the body to its natural state of alignment takes practice—and patience. As you learn the instructions in the following pages and begin to work with your child(ren), keep your reminders lighthearted rather than critical and nagging. Maintain a sense of humor. Adults who demonstrate a determination for improving their own alignment send a clear message that being naturally aligned is a worthwhile endeavor, in spite of the challenges involved, such as remembering to practice often. Children will respect you for this and will be more likely to be enthusiastically receptive.

Not only are you taking steps to improve your overall health by aligning your bones, you are using this practice to learn to be more present and mindful. Teaching these qualities to children is a valuable gift we give them. Once you and your child get the hang of this, you will understand how natural alignment becomes the gift that never stops giving.

PART TWO

PUPPET POSTURE

Guidelines & Instructions
for Children & Adults

A Few Words for Adults

Part Two is a guide for adults and children to work through together. While it is written with the older elementary student in mind, these instructions also work well for adults. Children will need to be guided through each one of these steps. You can begin by going through the first part of the book together, discussing the photographs and building interest in *why* it's important to learn how to align one's bones. It is also helpful to read through the instructions before introducing them to your child, depending on your child's level of interest and ability to understand the details.

While practicing the steps that follow, you'll be overriding longstanding patterns, so do keep in mind that some of what you and your child(ren) will be doing may feel strange at first. The more you understand these instructions in your own body, the more you'll be able to help guide a child through them, as well.

- Refer to the images in this book of aligned "puppets" and work to copy in your own body what you see in them, without creating any tension. Stop if you feel any discomfort or pain. Read through all the instructions and gently try again.
- If you are confused by the instructions, ask another adult to go through the steps with you. Two heads can be better than one in working with this. (Refer to the Appendix for teachers in your area.)
- Putting these rules into practice often feels "weird" at first. This makes sense, actually, because you are experiencing something that is different from your "norm".
- Use a mirror or digital camera to give yourselves feedback. Notice what you look and feel like with puppet strings pulling up on the front of your body, then loosened, and then attached to the back of your body.
- Don't give up! Even if it seems like a lot to remember, remind yourself that you are changing longstanding habits, and the strangeness of it will soon wear off.
- *FEEL* what you're doing. It's easy to fall into over-analyzing unfamiliar instructions, but once you understand the basic concepts, get out of your thinking mind and into your feeling body. Relax! You're going for greater ease and comfort, so let that be your guide.

A word about pain: Learn to distinguish between uncomfortable sensation. Ask your self if it's a pinch or a pull. A pinch, or sharp pain, should be avoided completely, but a pull is likely to be a stretching sensation in a muscle that has been too tight from overwork or a complaint from a muscle that has been on vacation for many years. As you pay close attention to these sensations, you'll learn to distinguish between them for yourself. Cultivate mindfulness inside your skin.

The following pages show how to sit, stand, bend. walk and sleep in natural ways. Presented in a larger font size so that children who are old enough will be able to read along, the instructions should be followed carefully, to be sure they are fully understood. The instructions start out with very simple language and descriptions, although they soon become more detailed and include words like "compression", as well as a number of anatomical terms. You may want to use this as an opportunity to help your child learn the meaning of new words and concepts.

Children are often unaccustomed to talking about their bodies or using them in an experiential way. If they are in a group setting, there may be a bit of nervous laughter or even outright silliness at first. Adults can help put children at ease by keeping things lighthearted and fun, while also emphasizing the value of getting to know oneself "inside your skin". Remind them that you are learning this right along with them and that you can each help guide one another through this experience. Children appreciate being partners in a process of mutual learning.

Once they begin to grasp the details of natural alignment, children typically respond with enthusiasm. The more you invite them to share their experiences of what they are learning and feeling in their bodies, the more they will want to participate.

These lessons are best learned in small segments. Once the information is learned, reminders can be interspersed and details reinforced throughout the day. The most effective approach seems to be short lessons that introduce bits of information that are later reviewed and built upon by subsequent segments. Each time you introduce new information, begin by spending a few minutes reviewing what has been covered up to that point. These instructions do take a bit of repetition to sink into the mind, as well as the body.

Most important, avoid criticizing or teasing children about any aspects of what they are doing. These lessons are only learned through encouragement and sharing, through words that demonstrate acceptance by you and foster self-acceptance by your child.

Have fun with this! The more relaxed you are, the more your body will respond and lead the way "home".

Four   Step-by-Step Instructions

Our Bodies and the Earth

The earth is a giant ball spinning in space. The reason we don't fall off, no matter what side of the earth we happen to be on, is because of **gravity.**

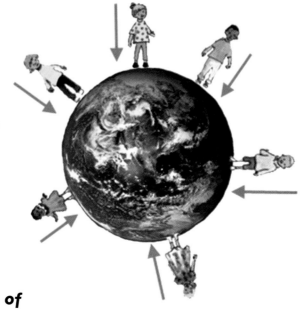

Gravity is a force that pulls all matter toward the center of the earth. This force pulls things to the earth along a straight line called the **vertical axis of gravity** or plumb line. (Vertical means straight up and down.)

You can see gravity working around you all the time. If you hold a solid object in your hand and then let go of it, it will fall straight to the ground along this vertical line. It doesn't fall sideways, and it doesn't fall up; it always falls straight down. This is gravity pulling the object down toward the center of the earth.

If you tie a string to a key and hold the end of the string, the key will hang straight down toward your feet. This is gravity at work, pulling the key toward the center of the earth.

This will work in just the same way even for someone standing on the other side of the world from you!

A scaffold is a **framework** of **vertical** posts (up and down) and **horizontal** poles (side to side) that are connected to each other at joints.

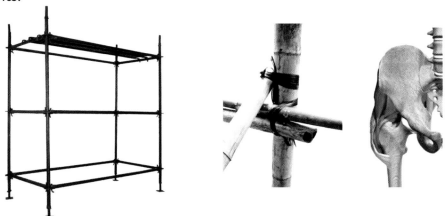

Your skeleton works like scaffolding, acting as the framework of support for your whole body. In some places, scaffolding is made of bamboo poles that are tied together with twine, like the tendons and ligaments that hold together your body's joints. Can you picture the stress caused to these joints if a vertical post is pulled off the center line? This same kind of stress is frequently put on human joints and is the cause of many problems people face, from injuring themselves playing sports, developing pain problems when they get older, or having hip replacement surgery.

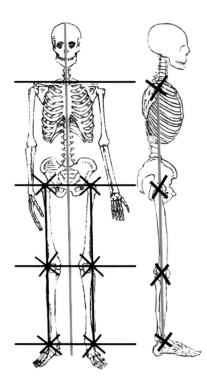

Unlike scaffolding, human joints are designed to bend and move. However, the "home base" of support for the bones is always a straight center line with each joint stacked up along the vertical axis of gravity.

These same rules apply to the "stacking" of the bones of your spine (vertebrae), as well as to the construction of buildings and everything else in the physical world.

How to Be a Happy Dog

Let's Pretend—just for now—

that you are a dog.

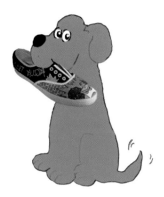

You're a happy little dog. Your family loves you and takes good care of you. You're so happy that you wag your tail a lot.

You love to chase balls and romp and play. Sometimes you get so excited that you forget the rules you've been taught.

In fact, one day you get so excited, you grab a brand new shoe from the porch and run outside to chew it. One of the people in your family catches you. "Bad Dog!" she scolds.

You feel terrible! You feel so bad you stop wagging your tail. Do you know what you do with your tail instead of wagging it?

That's right! You tuck your tail between your legs.

When dogs are happy, they wag their tails. Their backs are long and straight. The bones of the spine line up one on top of the other.

When dogs are sad, they tuck their tails under. Their backs are round, and the bones of the spine curl into a collapsed shape.

Do this yourself. What do you notice about your back when you "wag your tail"? What happens when you "tuck your tail"? What happens when you try to wag a tail that is "tucked" under?

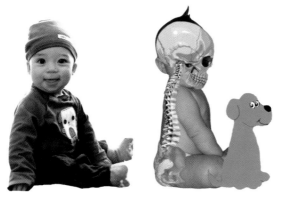

A baby's spine is long and tall, when he or she is sitting, because the spine is supported on a "wagging tail" pelvis.

Babies don't have tails, of course, but they do have a tailbone. Healthy babies who are old enough to sit up by themselves all "wag their tails". In other words, they sit as if their tailbones were reaching out behind them. In this way, healthy babies are "Happy Dogs".

Some children forget how to sit on a "wagging tail" pelvis and develop slouching habits that are not healthy. You might say they are being "Sad Dogs".

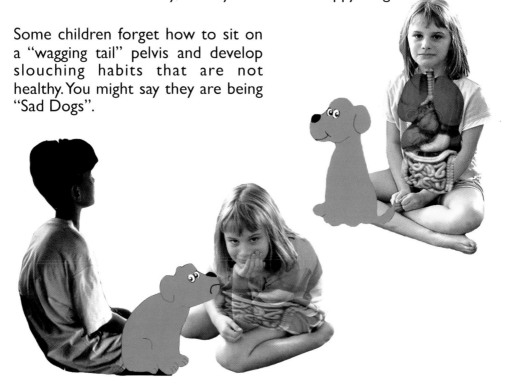

Tucking your "tail" under and collapsing the spine causes more than just aches and pains. Collapsing like this can affect your breathing, circulation of blood, digestion of food, and can interfere messages sent to and from your brain which pass through the spinal cord located in the center of your spine.

Finding Your Bones

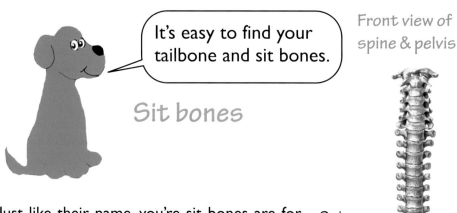

It's easy to find your tailbone and sit bones.

Sit bones

Just like their name, you're sit bones are for sitting. You can find your sit bones by sliding your right hand, palm facing up, under your right buttock or "butt". Roll around on your hand until you feel a pokey bone pressing into your fingers. This is your right "sit bone". You have another one just like it on the other side. Tuck your "tail" under and feel how the sit bone slides forward on your hand. "Wag your tail" and feel how it moves back. *This* is where it belongs.

Take hold of this bone and pull it out even further behind you. It can take time for the "wagging tail" muscles to get used to this, so be patient and keep doing this. Pretty soon, this won't feel strange anymore.

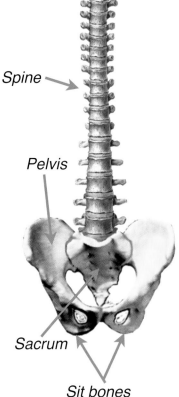

Front view of spine & pelvis

Spine →

Pelvis

Sacrum

Sit bones

Sitting on a wedge-shaped cushion or a towel or blanket folded to form a wedge is important for everyone learning how to "park the pelvis" and should be used whenever possible.

Caution: Be sure that you are not using muscle tension to "lift" the tailbone up behind you. Doing this will create tension in low back muscles and cause compression in your spine. Sit bones move straight out behind you and stay "parked" there.

Reach behind you and place your fingers on your back. Move your fingers up and down the center line and feel the bones of your spine. Do they form an even line all the way up your back or do some bones stick out or curve in more than others? Eventually, you will want this to be an even line.

Now walk your fingers further down your back, below your waist. At the bottom of the spine is the sacrum. Can you follow this bone with your fingers all the way to its pointy end? This is the tailbone or *coccyx* and, even though it curves in, it should feel like it is "wagging" behind you when you are sitting on the front edge of your sit bones.

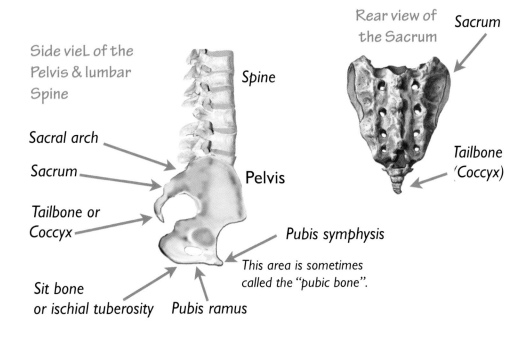

Side vieL of the
Pelvis & lumbar
Spine

Spine

Rear view of
the Sacrum

Sacrum

Sacral arch

Sacrum

Tailbone or
Coccyx

Pelvis

Tailbone
(Coccyx)

Pubis symphysis

This area is sometimes
called the "pubic bone".

Sit bone
or ischial tuberosity

Pubis ramus

Remember how your back rounded when you were being scolded and you tucked your "tail" between your legs?

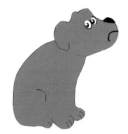

With your sit bones out behind you, your weight will shift onto the front of the pelvis. This "Happy Dog" foundation makes it possible to support a long, healthy spine.

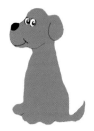

When you were a baby and a toddler, you were always "wagging your tail".

Meet Mindful Dog

Mindful Dog is like your best friend. Mindful Dog is a part of you that helps you remember to pay attention to yourself—what you are feeling inside your skin and what you are thinking and doing—right here and right now. When you see this picture of Mindful Dog beaming out at you from the page, you can ask yourself these questions: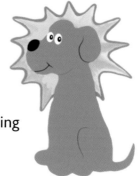

❖ Are my bones aligned? (You'll be learning how to do this very soon!)

❖ Am I breathing?

❖ What does it feel like to breathe?

❖ Where do I feel the breath touching inside my body?
 ❖ Do my lower ribs widen?
 ❖ Can I feel the breath touching and widening my back?

❖ Am I feeling relaxed or tense?

❖ If there is tension in me, where is it? What does it feel like?

❖ What can I do to let the tension go?
 ❖ Does aligning my bones help?
 ❖ Does imagining the breath gently rising up from deep inside and then softly dropping away help me to relax?

It takes patience to go through these questions. Pretty soon, though, you'll learn how to ask—and answer—these questions more easily. You'll learn how to relax without collapsing, because once your bones are doing the job they are supposed to do—holding you up—it's safe for you to relax! It feels GREAT!

First you ALIGN, then you RELAX!

First You Align, Then You Relax

First, you align means that you begin by finding the underlying support of your bones that makes it possible to let go of unnecessary tension. In other words, you let aligned bones do the job of holding you up instead of relying on struggling muscles to do it.

This all sounds simple enough, but *how,* exactly, do you do this, especially when you are sitting or standing up? How do you align your bones so that you can be easily upright? The pages that follow will show you how to find the support from your bones so that you can be upright *and* relaxed.

You'll soon learn how to rediscover the "center line of gravity"—or "plumb line"—within yourself. Remember, this is what you first learned as a toddler when you figured out how to stand and walk without falling over. It was not just muscle tension that held you up but discovering out how to balance in the center, much like learning to ride a bicycle. Once you re-learn how to be aligned along this center line, it will be important to practice by paying attention to how you sit, stand, bend, walk, and sleep. When your organs and other parts of your body are aligned around this center line, you will find that it will be surprisingly comfortable to sit up or stand for longer periods without having to worry about collapsing or using tension to hold yourself up. Misalignment of the skeleton is why we slouch and is the cause of much of the pain and discomfort millions of people experience on a daily basis.

Learning to be supported by aligned bones is made easy by imagining that you are a puppet controlled by strings from above. This kind of puppet is called a **marionette**, and the person who controls the strings is a **puppeteer.**

You are the Puppet and the Puppeteer!

It's not some outside force that's pulling your strings; it's your own mind that is doing it. This means you are the one in charge whenever you decide to pay attention to yourself in this way. It can feel good to know you have this kind of control over yourself and how you feel.

Imagine yourself as a puppet held by strings attached to the back of your body. An imaginary puppeteer stands behind you, gently drawing these strings back and up, with just enough "tension" in the strings to support you from above. At the same time, you "hang" solidly from the strings, weighted and connected to the ground below you. This balance between dropping into the earth and rising up at the same time helps us learn how to experience our bodies in a natural way, without having to use too much effort or to worry about collapsing.

Imagining the support of puppet strings is a helpful way to re-learn how to stand, walk, sit, bend over, lift heavy things, reach for something on a high shelf, even sleep, in ways that keep you strong, healthy and comfortable. The following pages will show you in greater detail just how to use these imaginary puppet strings for greater ease and comfort. as well as genuine strength in all that you do.

Sitting Like a Happy Puppet

Learning how to sit with the support of imaginary puppet strings comes as a big relief to anyone who has a hard time knowing how to sit comfortably for long periods of time.

It's important to know how to sit upright without leaning back, since backrests are not always available. Sitting this way also re-teaches the body how to be self-supporting in any situation. You'll also learn how to make good use of a backrest when you have one, since leaning back is a great way to lengthen out your back.

Notice how, in all the examples below, the pelvis is in the "Happy Dog" position, and each spine is long and fully lengthened.

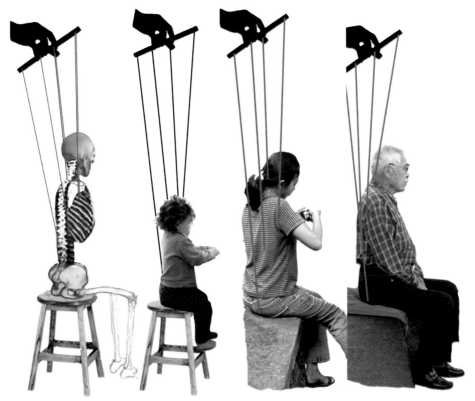

92 years old!

You will soon learn how to sit like a "Happy Puppet", but before you do, let's learn a bit more about sitting.

A Few Facts About Sitting

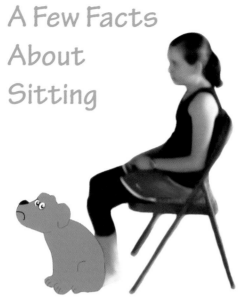

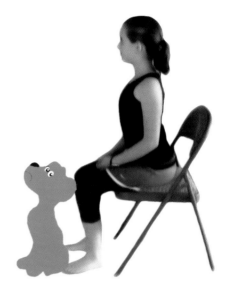

This is the way many people sit. The tailbone is tucked under, and the spine is rounded and collapsed. We think of this as "relaxing", but some muscles have to strain and work when our bones are not giving us support.

If you try to sit up "straight", you might do it like this, lifting your chest up, pulling your shoulders back and lifting your chin. It takes a lot of muscular effort to sit this way. Even the dog thinks so!

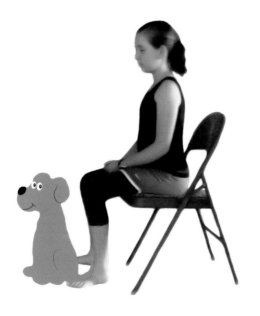

When you sit the same way you sat as a baby, your weight is on the front of your sit bones and your spine supports itself like the trunk of a tree. Sitting like this is easy and comfortable, once you re-learn how to do it. It takes practice to sit this way, so it's important to remember to pay attention.

Sitting Skeletons

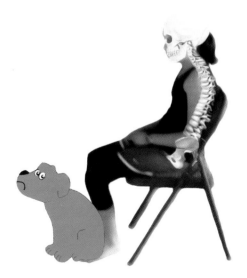

This is what is happening to your spine and to the spinal cord inside the spine when you sit like a "Sad Dog".

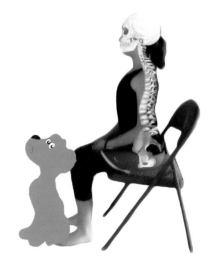

Even though the tailbone is back now, the chest is lifted up ,and the spine is overly curvy. Muscles are working too hard here.

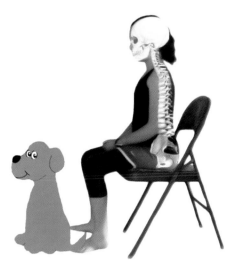

The chest is neither collapsed nor lifted up here. With the tailbone parked in "Happy Dog" mode, the spine is also straight.

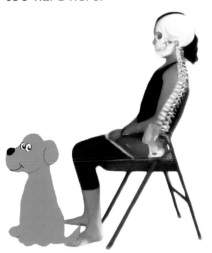

You will soon learn how to lean back in a chair, not by bending in the spine, but by lengthening the spine the way it is pictured here.

Where Puppet Strings Attach

The green dots mark the points where imaginary puppet strings attach at the back of your body. Knowing how to engage these strings will help you rediscover how to be supported by your bones.

Each point has two strings attached, one on the left and one on the right, except for the base of the skull, which has just one string attached at its base.

Remember that each step builds on top of the one below it. Be sure that you do not undo any steps when you put the next ones into action.

The five steps are as follows:

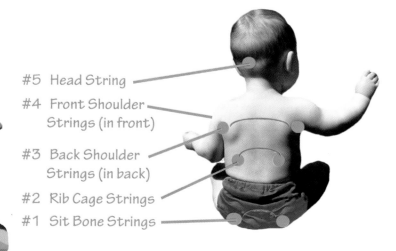

#5 Head String

#4 Front Shoulder Strings (in front)

#3 Back Shoulder Strings (in back)

#2 Rib Cage Strings

#1 Sit Bone Strings

These points are listed backwards, because the steps start from the bottom and work up to the top, the same way a building is built—from the ground up.

Sit Like a Puppet — It's Easy!
Five Simple Steps

All it takes are five simple steps to take you from sitting like this . . .

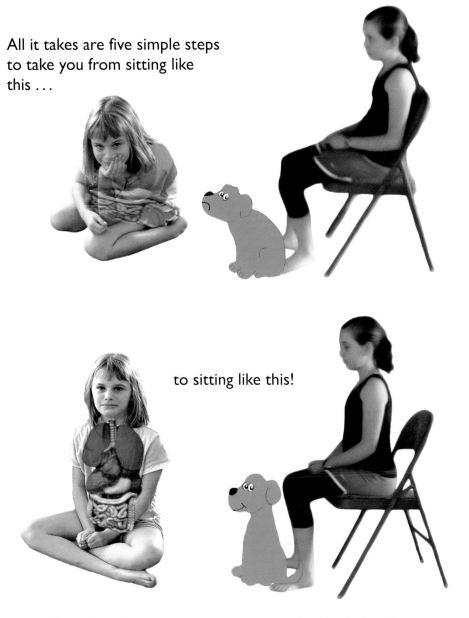

to sitting like this!

Note: *The 5 Easy Steps are presented on the left side of the following pages. Further information, for those "Who Want to Know More," is found on facing pages.*

Step #1: Sit Bone Strings —
Also called "Park Your Pelvis"

"Walk" your sit bones back

Sit with your feet flat on the floor about eighteen inches apart. Place your knees directly above your ankles and aim your knees out, away from each other.

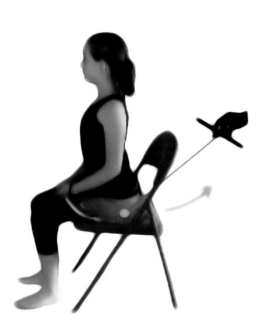

Lean to the left, shifting your weight onto your left sit bone. Imagine a puppet string attached to your right sit bone and "walk" the sit bone back behind you. Now lean to the right and walk the left sit bone back. Sense your weight on the front edge of your sit bones as the entire pelvic bone drops forward.

This is the same thing you did when you moved the sit bones back with your hand, but now you know how to do this in public!

Did your chest lift up when you did this? You don't want to arch your back like the picture above. If you automatically lift your chest when you set your weight on the front edge of your sit bones, Step #2 will show you how to correct this. You might think that pushing your chest out in front makes you sit up taller, but it actually compresses the spine in back, tightens the neck and causes tension in many muscles. Step #2 will show you how to remove the arch from your lower back.

DO NOT "lift" your sit bones up behind you by tightening muscles in your hips and back. Let the imaginary puppet strings draw them straight back, where they just "hang", as if weighted, from the strings above. If your back hurts when you do this, read through all the steps before proceeding with caution.

Know More about Step #1

This step sets the foundational position of the pelvis.

"Tucking the tail" (Sad Dog) is the most common instruction given by many to correct swayback (or lordosis) but doing this prevents the pelvis from supporting the spine. Arching in the lower back is almost always the result of a lifted rib cage, which must then be held in place with muscle tension.

A tucked-under or "Sad Dog" pelvis brings the sit bones forward and causes the pubic bone to curl up toward the navel. The spine loses its foundation of support and collapses into a rounded heap.

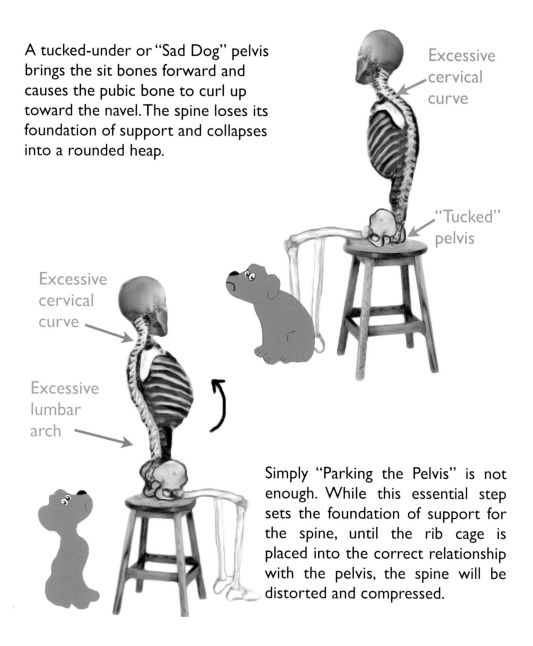

Excessive cervical curve

"Tucked" pelvis

Excessive cervical curve

Excessive lumbar arch

Simply "Parking the Pelvis" is not enough. While this essential step sets the foundation of support for the spine, until the rib cage is placed into the correct relationship with the pelvis, the spine will be distorted and compressed.

Step #2 Rib Cage Strings —

Also called "Hug a Tree"

Open your lower back

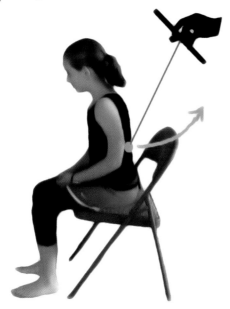

Wrap your hands around your middle, just above your waist. Roll your thumbs around to feel your lower ribs. Imagine puppet strings attached under each thumb, close to the bottom of the rib cage.

Without undoing Step #1 (in other words, keep your pelvis parked!), let the points under your thumbs reach toward the wall behind you. Do this slowly so that you can feel your lower back widen and fill out.

It's okay if this causes you to feel like you're slouching and your shoulders are dropping forward. The steps that follow will take care of this. You can also bring your arms in front of you and pretend you are hugging a very big tree, or wrap your arms around your shoulders and hug yourself! With your arms wrapped around your chest, drop your chin and lower your elbows toward the floor. This is another way to widen and open up your lower back. Can you feel it?

Don't worry about your shoulders. They will be fixed in Step #4. For now, you are just focused on making your lower back as long and wide as you can and enjoying the sensations that come with this. If you feel slouched, this is a positive sign that you are on the right track. This will be fixed in the following steps.

Know More about Step #2

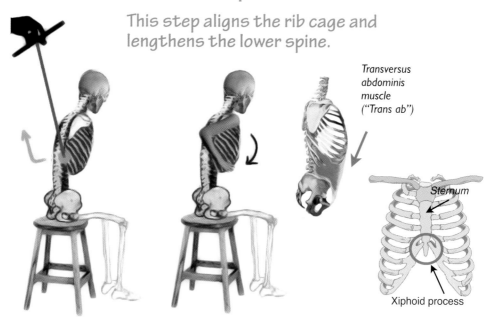

This step aligns the rib cage and lengthens the lower spine.

Transversus abdominis muscle ("Trans ab")

Sternum

Xiphoid process

"Tucking" the bottom front ribs in and up is another way to experience the action of the rib cage puppet strings. This is not the same as sucking in the belly or having "six-pack abs", an action that causes tension around the spine and disrupts the ability of the *obliques* and the deep *transversus abdominis* muscles to stabilize the torso. The "trans ab" muscle has horizontal fibers that are specifically designed to act as a deep inner corset. Located at the bottom of the breastbone (*sternum*) is an arrow-shaped point called the *xiphoid process* (pronounced zy-foid). This tip made of cartilage is a useful landmark to use for anchoring the rib cage and engaging your "core center." Imagine the xiphoid process sliding back and up, toward the middle of your back. With practice, you will feel your entire waist firming as you do this, as your torso narrows and lengthens. Be sure that you DO NOT let the distance between your pubic bone and navel grow shorter.

RELAXING UNNECESSARY TENSION IN THE BELLY:

Exaggerate the tension in your belly by pulling in your navel and holding it. Notice that you've stopped breathing. Pull it in even more and notice all the tension it takes to hold it. Now, let it out just a little bit . . . and a little bit more . . . and a little bit more . . . Keep going. It takes a bit of practice, but, before long, your abdomen will be more relaxed—and stronger. You might worry that your "abs" will get too loose, but the following steps will work to build the right kind of strength in the "core" or deepest abdominal muscles. Superficial tension in the belly prevents these muscles from being able to do their job. (Also see Chapter 5: Exercises.)

Step #3 Back Shoulder Strings —
Also called "Climb a Ladder"

Wiggle your armpits up to the sky.

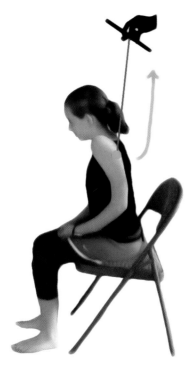

Imagine puppet strings just inside the back of each armpit. These strings lift the shoulders up toward your ears. Keep wiggling each armpit even higher, as this will lengthen your spine even more.

Don't worry about your lifted shoulders. Step #4 will put them where they belong. For now, just think about lengthening your spine upward along your back. This takes pressure off a compressed spine, intervertebral discs and nerve roots.

As you lengthen upward, muscles along your back and throughout your torso are also lengthened. You'll soon be gaining new strength in deep abdominal muscles that will help support a longer, more supple spine.

Helpful Tip:

Think of your torso as an elevator shaft with two elevators—one traveling up and the other traveling down at the same time. The "down" elevator travels down along the front of your body, taking the front of the pelvis into the "basement". This anchors the pelvis into the chair, as the floor of the pelvis widens and the *pubis symphysis* grows roots into the earth. The "up" elevator travels along the back of your body, taking the back of the armpits and the base of the skull up to the sky behind you. Both elevators are very wide, filling out the torso from side to side, as wide as possible. **Do not** lift your chest, even a little, as this will shorten and narrow your back. All the lengthening that is taking place is deep within the center of the spine.

Do you feel "new" muscles working in your abdomen?

Relax—and remember to breathe!

Know More about Step #3

This step lengthens the upper spine.

The pelvis forms a tripod of support made up of the two sit bones and the *pubis*. Keeping the pelvis deeply rooted into the seat makes it possible for the spine to lengthen upward, along the back (one elevator up, the other one down).

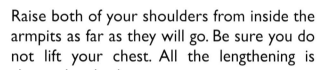

Raise both of your shoulders from inside the armpits as far as they will go. Be sure you do not lift your chest. All the lengthening is along the back at this point. Watch your breath gently rising and falling. Can you feel the breath touching your entire back and the sides of your rib cage? The point here is to fully lengthen the upper spine. For now, your shoulders will be lifted up around your ears.

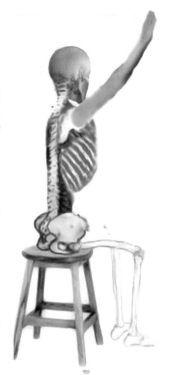

Another way you can cultivate length in your spine is to raise your arms as if trying to

It's important that both Step #1 (Sit Bone Strings) and Step #2 (Rib Cage Strings) remain fully engaged. Remember that each new step builds on the one below it, working from the bottom up.

The next step will take care of your raised up shoulders.

Step #4 Front Shoulder Strings —
Also called "Putting on the Saddle"

Circle the front of your armpits forward, up and way back.

This set of strings attaches just inside the **front** of each armpit and places the shoulders squarely on top of the rib cage. **Do this, one side at a time,** until you are able to keep your chest from pushing forward when you do both sides together.

The green arrow shows how each puppet string rolls up, around and then way back. Your elbow extends behind you, close to the waist, to get your shoulder squarely on top of the rib cage. Do not pull your shoulders down. Let each one sit like a saddle straddling both sides of the rib cage. This action helps "snap" the entire upper body into a solid, stable position. Your elbows will rest near the back of your waist.

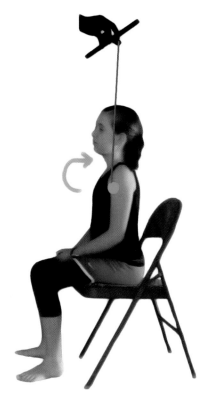

It is common for this to feel "weird" at first, especially if your shoulders habitually fall forward. As muscles around your shoulders adjust over time, this will feel more familiar.

These strings open the front of the body in a wholly natural way and create width between the shoulders.

Reminder: As long as all the previous steps remain in effect and the pelvis is deeply rooted, the entire upper body opens, front to back and side to side in an equal and balanced way.

72

Know More about Step #4

This step widens the upper torso and stabilizes the shoulder on top of the rib cage

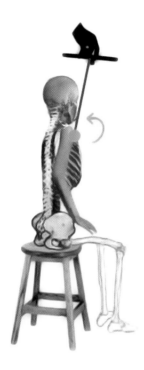

Don't let the breastbone (*sternum*) push forward while doing this step. Maintain length and width through the upper body in an equal and balanced way. Engaging wide "elevators" (Page 68) front to back and side to side, helps with this. This step also opens the "gate" for the cervical spine to rise up through the neck so your head can delicately balance on top. The head balances delicately on top of a long, rising spine. Picture each shoulder blade as a hand on your back and sense the "heel of the hand" gently pressing into your rib cage. This helps "snap" the saddle-like features of the shoulder girdle into place. Again, do not lift the breastbone when doing this.

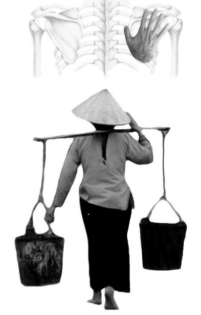

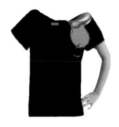
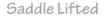
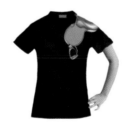
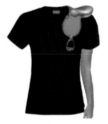

Saddle Lifted   Saddle Dropped   Saddle Aligned

If you think of the top of the shoulder as the back of a horse, an aligned shoulder sits like a saddle right on top of the horse. This position provides stability for the whole upper frame.

Step #5 Head String —

Also called "Be a Puppet"

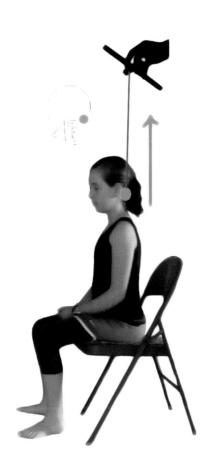

Once you have built the foundation through the first four steps, you may still need to set the position of your head. You do this by imagining a puppet string attached at the base of the skull, at the point where the skull rounds inward toward the spine at the top of your neck. You can feel this "dip" at the bottom of your skull with your fingers. This is called the *occiput.*

This puppet string attachment is very delicate, almost more a thought than an action. Sense the base of the skull rising upward (as softly as rising bread dough) as the back of your neck widens and lengthens. Be sure that you are not creating any tension and that your neck muscles are completely relaxed.

You might feel, at first, like you are having to look down at the floor in front of you, which is very common. If this is the case, relax your belly, open your eyes wider to look forward and relax. As you stay anchored in aligned bones, continue to imagine the neck lengthening. You will be looking at the world with your eyes more wide open!

Relax, relax, relax! Don't "hold" this final sitting position stiffly. You want to feel solid and anchored (through aligned bones) but also loose and fluid (relaxed, elastic muscles).

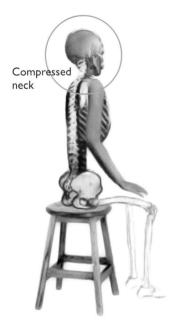

Compressed neck

The base of the skull hangs delicately from this top string, an invitation for the back of the neck to elongate. There is also a gentle drop of the chin toward the chest. Visualize your neck muscles softening as you exhale slowly. When you exhale, feel the back of the neck also growing wide.

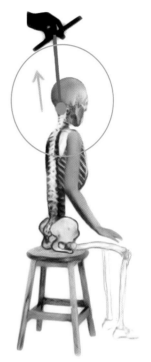

Long, Relaxed Neck

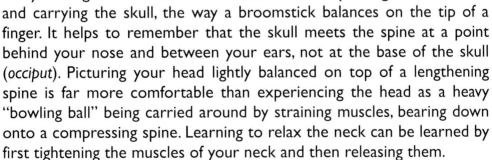

Bring awareness to the spot at the front of the throat where one might have an "Adam's Apple". Imagine this spot floating softly toward the back of your throat, then sense it rising up the back of your neck like a helium-filled balloon. Make this the softest action possible. As you imagine the front of your throat floating backwards, sense the spine rising softly through the center of the neck, effortlessly lifting and carrying the skull, the way a broomstick balances on the tip of a finger. It helps to remember that the skull meets the spine at a point behind your nose and between your ears, not at the base of the skull (*occiput*). Picturing your head lightly balanced on top of a lengthening spine is far more comfortable than experiencing the head as a heavy "bowling ball" being carried around by straining muscles, bearing down onto a compressing spine. Learning to relax the neck can be learned by first tightening the muscles of your neck and then releasing them.

Putting It All Together — Summary of Steps

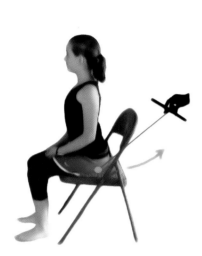

#1 Sit Bone Strings
"Walk" your sit bones back.
Parks the pelvis

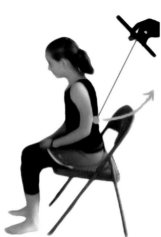

#2 Rib Cage Strings
Extend your lower ribs behind you.
Opens the lower back

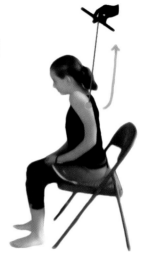

#3 Back Shoulder Strings
Wiggle your armpits up to the sky.
Lengthens the spine

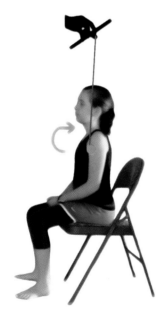

#4 Front Shoulder Strings
Circle the front of your armpits up and back.
Places the shoulder "saddle"

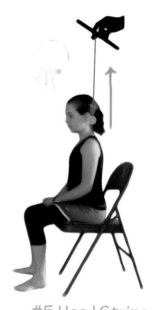

#5 Head String
Sense the base of the skull rising upward.
Lengthens the neck, balances the head

Lean Back in a Chair

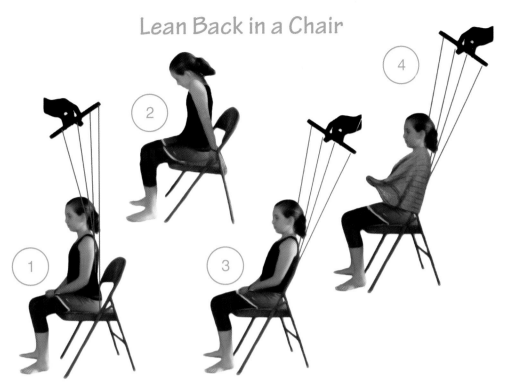

Be sure the Sit Bone Strings are drawn behind you (in other words, keep your pelvis firmly "parked"). Keep the pubic bone connected to the chair as you use your hands on the seat or the sides of your chair to lift the middle of your back up onto an imaginary shelf high up behind you. (Do NOT arch your back or push your chest forward as you lean back. Rather the front of the body moves into the back.) Rest your lengthened back onto the back rest. Notice how this creates a shortcut for engaging the puppet strings and "tucking up" the front of the rib cage. (Step #2). In fact, now that you know where the puppet strings attach, you can use this shortcut for "tucking and lifting" the rib cage in any position you find yourself in. This draws the bottom of your rib cage up and away from your pelvis and lengthens out your spine. Focus on all the strings keeping your back wide and long, as if you were wrapping a shawl around your shoulders and meeting the shawl with the fullness of your back. This may feel a bit like you are rounding your back.

Now, without changing anything, let your shoulders, one at a time, slide back onto the top of the rib cage (Saddle the horse—Step #4).

Finally, relax your weight down into the chair, noticing that you do not collapse and that your spine remains nicely lengthened. It is safe to relax when your bones are aligned.

How Sitting, Standing and Bending are the Same

Although the spine acts as the "trunk of the tree", it is not rigid or stiff and remains fluid in its movements. This does not mean, however, that we are meant to bend in the spine. The main function of the spinal joints is to provide fluidity of movement and shock absorption. These joints (*facets*) exist between each bone of the spine (*vertebra*). A small pillow like structure (intervertebral disc) provides cushioning between each bone, as well as shock absorption whenever you move.

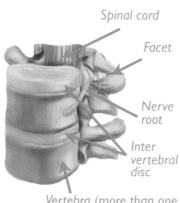

Spinal cord

Facet

Nerve root

Inter vertebral disc

Vertebra (more than one are "vertebrae")

Bending takes place at the hip and knee joints. The pelvis rotates over the thigh bone (*femur*), while the spine stays intact (See red boxes below). In this way, the system of muscles and bones (pulleys and levers) functions a bit like a building crane. It's important to move according to nature's design. People who move naturally experience fewer aches and pains and are less likely to be injured. Notice that all the children's spines, pictured below, remain fully lengthened whether they are sitting, standing or bending.

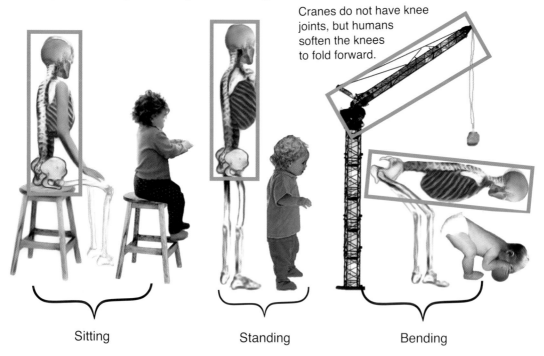

Cranes do not have knee joints, but humans soften the knees to fold forward.

Sitting

Standing

Bending

Folding forward at the hips

All natural bending takes place in the hip joints, deep inside the crease where the front of the legs meets the torso. Babies figure this out as they are learning how to sit up and balance on the *pubis ramus* and sit bones, in an upright position.

Imagine again that a string is attached to each sit bone. Notice that when you think of these strings being drawn out behind you, you begin to fold forward at the hips. The more the strings are pulled back, the more you bend forward. Like the crane pictured on the facing page, babies do not bend along the spine when they bend forward. Natural bending always maintains the full length of the spine.

Many people bend the spine while engaging in daily activities and exercise routines. Not o n l y does this tuck the tailbone, it causes compression of spinal discs. Doing this often trains unhealthy habits into the body's "muscle memory" and contributes to many of the serious degenerative conditions that people develop as they grow older.

Pay attention to keeping your spine long and your back wide in all your daily activities, even yoga practices. If the muscles in the back of your thighs (hamstrings) are too tight when you bend forward for you to keep your spine straight, bend your knees. Don't sacrifice the integrity of your spine just to stretch your hamstrings. There are safe ways to lengthen the hamstrings (see Chapter 5) and over time, these muscles will lengthen naturally as you learn how to re-inhabit your body in a natural way.

Getting Up from a Chair

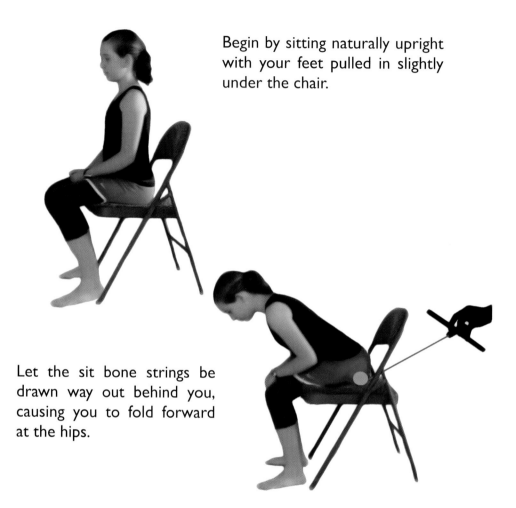

Begin by sitting naturally upright with your feet pulled in slightly under the chair.

Let the sit bone strings be drawn way out behind you, causing you to fold forward at the hips.

Now, let yourself "fall" forward as the sit bone strings are pulled swiftly out behind you. The pull of the strings is strong enough to raise your buttocks off the seat slightly, while your weight shifts entirely onto both feet. Press your feet deeply into the floor as your knees aim wide, out over your pinky toes.

Repeat this a few more times, rocking back and forth to bring your sit bones off the chair. DO NOT engage any muscles in your back or neck while doing this, but rely on leg muscles instead. Puppet strings in all the right places keep your back wide and long. This helps to create a forward momentum that brings your sit bones off the chair and your weight fully onto your feet.

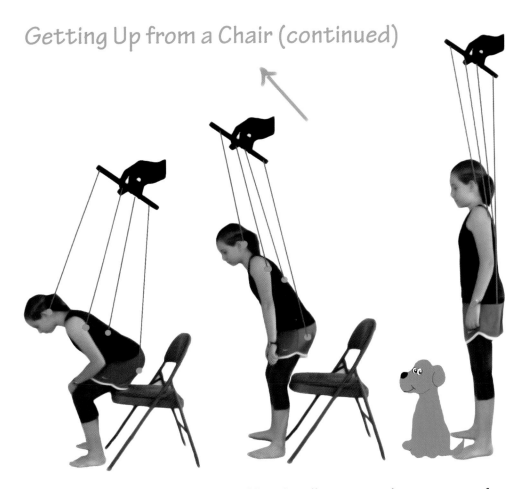

Once you've gotten the hang of "rocking" your weight onto your feet, press your feet deep into the floor and let the strength of your legs bring you to standing. Doing this often will strengthen your legs in a fully balanced way, prevent your back and neck muscles from working unnecessarily, and protect the length of your spine.

The puppet strings stabilize your spine, keeping it straight as you do this. All the strings along the back of your body are gently drawn forward and up at the same time. No one string is pulled more than another; they all work together to bring you out of the chair and into a standing position.

Any and all bending takes place in the hips and knees, nowhere else. Strong legs provide support for a solid, stable structure above.

Strong legs bring you up to standing.

Bending

Bending forward from a standing position is a bit different from getting out of a chair, because, rather than beginning with knees that are already bent, the knees must now bend from a straightened position.

To do this, imagine strings attached to the front of each knee. These strings are drawn forward at the same time the sit bone strings are drawn back. This causes the knees and hips to bend simultaneously. It's all one easy action. The knee strings also draw out to the outside, aiming the knees over the pinky toes.

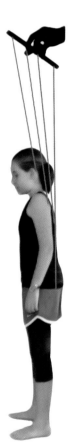

If you watch babies and toddlers, you will see that this is how they bend. They do not bend forward with locked knees. Bending *always* begins with your "butt" moving back, your knees bending out at the same time, and your back remaining straight.

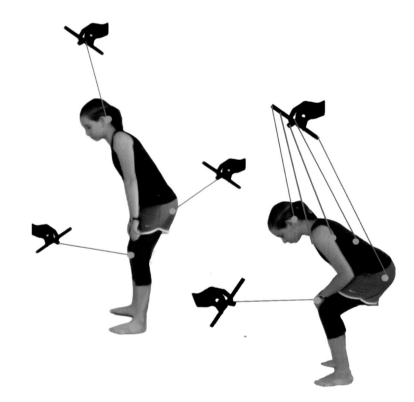

Bending (continued)

To bend even further, so that you can pick up something from the floor, bend the knees and hips even more. This will keep the spine long, rather than giving in to the common tendency to round the back while bending further.

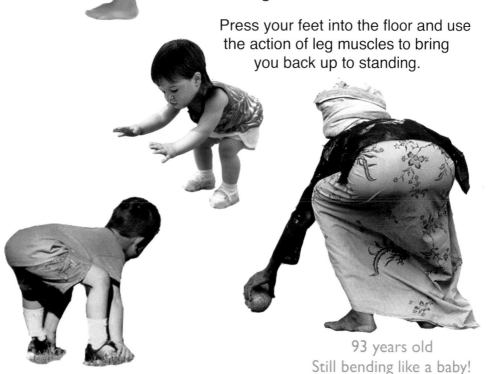

Babies and toddlers never lock their knees when they bend forward, always bending their knees, instead. To bend more deeply, the often raise the sit bones higher. Bending this way, when done frequently, builds natural, balanced strength in the muscles of the legs and helps to develop strong arches in the feet.

Bending like this will give you all the flexibility you will ever need. You'll remain easily flexible, even into old age.

Press your feet into the floor and use the action of leg muscles to bring you back up to standing.

93 years old
Still bending like a baby!

Sit Back Down

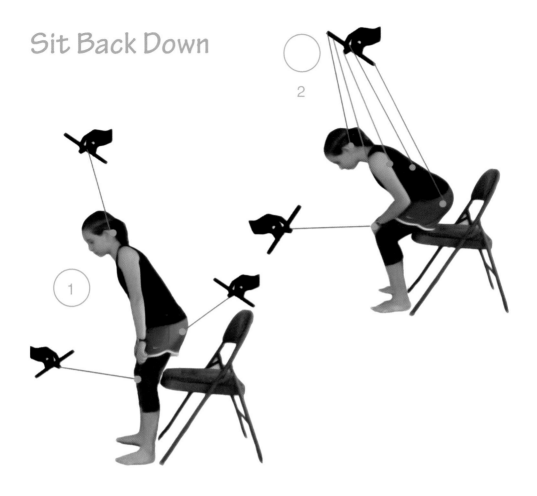

Stand in front of a chair with the backs of your legs barely touching the edge of the seat. Bend forward by engaging the sit bone and knee strings at the same time.

As you begin to bend down, make sure everything above your hips moves as one unit. Your back remains wide and filled out. Use the imaginary puppet strings to help you do this. Do not lift your chin. The head string will keep your neck long, while your chin drops slightly toward your chest.

Your sit bones extend behind you like a wagging tail as you use the strength of your bending legs to slowly lower your pelvis closer to the chair. Remember to keep your knees aiming wide.

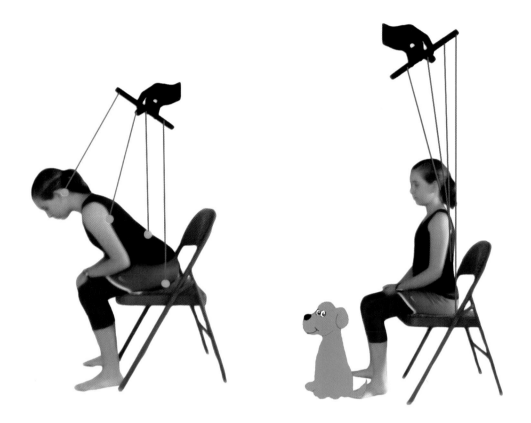

Picture your weight being placed onto the very front edge of your pelvis (or pubic bone) as it comes into contact with the seat. This will help to "park your pelvis" before you come up to sitting.

Important! Do not let old habits, such as lifting your chest or your chin, bring you up to sitting. Instead, pause for a moment while still folded forward, and then imagine the rib cage, shoulder and head strings working to widen and lengthen your entire back, as they help to draw you up to a sitting position. (This is like "spreading the shawl" across your back when leaning back in the chair, only now you are coming to an upright position.) If your shoulders are lifted or rolled forward when you come up to sitting, use the strings at the front of the shoulders, one at a time, to place them on top of the rib cage.

Standing

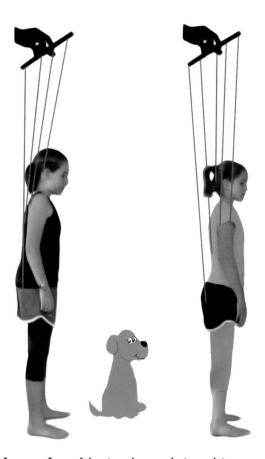

Look down at the tops of your feet. Notice how doing this moves your thighs and sit bones back and lines up your legs along the vertical axis. You have also shifted your weight more onto your heels, where it belongs. Let the puppet strings on your back and under your shoulders widen and lengthen your entire back. Take time to feel the effect of each step along the way. Place your shoulder "saddles" on top of the rib cage, then, let your head hang from the puppet string at the base of your skull. The front of your throat floats toward the back of your neck. Relax. This may feel a little "odd" at first, but as you practice this, it will become more familiar.

Imagining the support of puppet strings helps distribute your weight through an aligned skeleton. This "parks the pelvis" in the position that supports the spine and keeps the back long and wide, with equal length and width across the front of the body, too. Standing with such balanced distribution of the body's weight makes it possible to stand comfortably for long periods of time. **DO NOT "lift" your sit bones**; once they have moved back, simply let them hang from the puppet strings above.

What aligned standing looks like

Legs as pillars of support

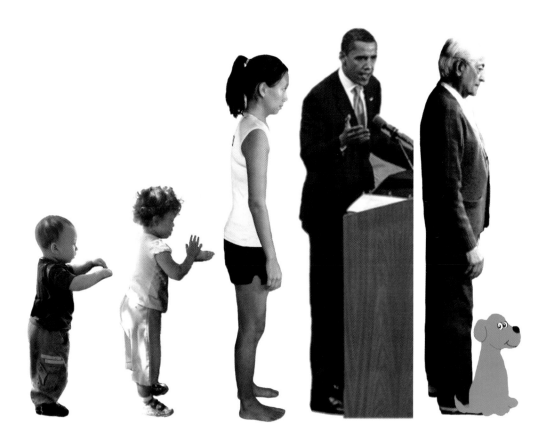

Babies and toddlers set the example of what aligned standing looks like, supported on two solid legs with fully lengthened spines. Adults who never lose this alignment are good role models, demonstrating that, as you get older, you can still be upright and relaxed. The man on the far right, Jiddu Krishnamurti, was 85 years old when this photo was taken, clearly demonstrating that a lifetime of support from aligned bones can lead to a "youthful" kind of old age. This is far different from many older people whose bodies only become more and more collapsed and stiff as the years go by. It's important to develop these habits when you are young, because it is harder to release stiff, tense muscles when you are older.

Walking

Stand naturally, as you have just learned to do. Decide which foot will take the first step. As the puppet strings begin to draw you forward in the direction of the green arrow, you will have to take a step so as not to fall face first. This begins a forward momentum; give yourself over to it. Be sure your weight lands on your heel, although it may be shared by the front of the medial arch. Your front knee is aiming toward your pinky toe and is ever-so-slightly bent and soft as you land on your foot. Notice your weight landing more on the outside than the inside of your foot, especially if you have a tendency to roll your ankles inward (pronation) and have low or collapsed arches. The toes of your back foot help to propel you forward.

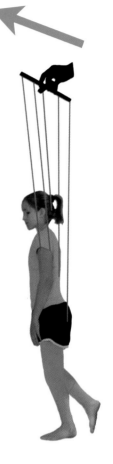

Your head and shoulders lead ahead of your hips and pelvis, your sit bones are extended behind you, and your spine is long and open. Let the puppet strings move you along and be sure the back of your neck is long and wide, hanging ever so gently from the puppet string, at the base of the skull, that is helping to draw you forward.

DO NOT actively lift up your tailbone or sit bones, as this will cause tension in your lower back. Your back muscles should feel more relaxed now that your legs and buttock muscles are doing the job of transporting your body.

Walking with the help of puppet strings puts the action into the feet, legs and buttocks, where it belongs. See if you can sense muscles in your buttocks (*gluteus*) working to move you along, like hands gently pushing you forward. You can even place your hands on your buttocks and feel them working as you walk.

Try not to think too much about what you're doing so much as just letting yourself be moved forward by the puppet strings in the direction of the green arrow above. This will override unhelpful patterns or "default settings" that are already in place and can be difficult to overcome.

What relaxed walking looks like

People whose skeletons are naturally aligned all have the same relaxed, graceful appearance when walking. Even carrying heavy loads on their heads is done with grace and ease of movement. This is because aligned bones are carrying the weight of the load, and an aligned, supple spine rises upwards from below, rather than being compressed down from above. The chest is not lifted but is broad and wide, as is the upper back.

The head leads, creating a forward momentum that is effortless, while the weight comes down fully onto the front leg. This leg is *under* the body, not extended out in front of it. The knee, which is slightly bent and tracks to the outside, acts as a shock absorber, protecting joints throughout the body. The toes of the back foot play an active role in propelling the body forward, as they gently grasp the ground and push off from behind.

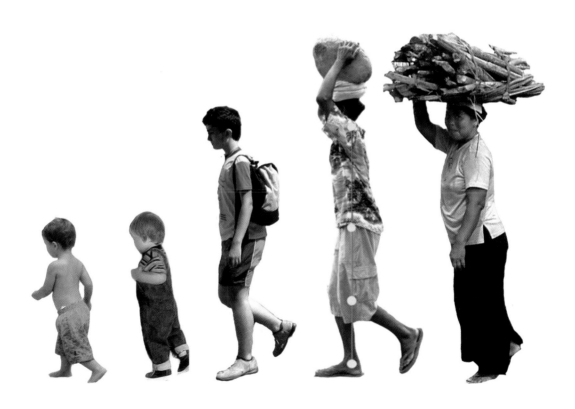

Resting / Sleeping
on your back

Sit in front of two soft pillows with your knees bent.

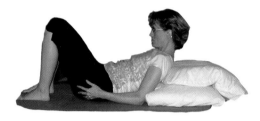

As you begin to lie back, press both elbows into the floor and sense puppet strings being pulled up behind you. Your entire back is carefully laid out as long and wide as possible, one vertebra at a time, across the surface on which you are lying (Spread the shawl, Steps #2 & #3). The lower edge of the first pillow will come to the bottom of your shoulder blades, and the pillow on top comes just under the top edge of your shoulders.

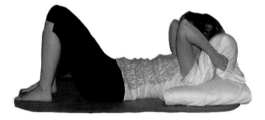

Do NOT tuck your tailbone under. Puppet strings draw your sit bones behind you (Step #1). You can place a pillow under your knees if you wish.

If necessary, reach up with both hands and roll the top pillow under to support a fully lengthened neck. You can also use your hands on the base of the skull to lengthen your neck further (Step #5). Be sure that your chin is not too close to your chest and that the throat remains soft and open.

As you "saddle up" your shoulders, feel your shoulder blades slide down your back (Step #4), as your arms come to rest at your sides.

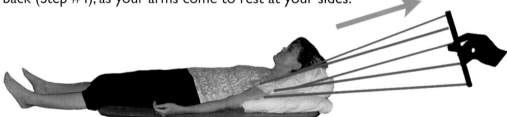

As muscles deep inside begin to relax and lengthen, you will be able to eventually lower or remove the top pillow. For now, however, using two pillows will assist in releasing the tension in small deep muscles that cause the back to arch and prevent full opening of the spine. Again, if your low back is arching or feels tight place a pillow under your knees, but DO NOT tuck your butt under.
Breathe—and focus on the exhalation as an opportunity to "melt" the back of your body, long and wide.

Resting / Sleeping
on your side

Lie on your side with one pillow (or two, if needed) under your head so that your head is supported in a neutral position. This is the same position, relative to your body, as if you were sitting or standing—neither too high, nor too low.

Bring the bottom of the pillow(s) snugly to the top of your lower shoulder to fully support your neck. Bend your knees slightly.

Press into the floor with the hand of your upper arm and raise your hips just enough to draw your sit bones out behind you as you "park your pelvis" (Step #1). In other words, scoot your pubic bone behind you.

Take hold of the pillow and draw it (and your head) toward your knees, as the rib cage strings draw the bottom of your ribs back (Step #2).

Scoot your lower armpit (the one on the floor) in a straight line, further away from your hips (Step #3). Feel your spine lengthen as you do this. This traction of the spine can be repeated again after a few minutes as muscles relax and the spine is able to lengthen more. Do not undo Steps # 1 or #2 above.

Rest the elbow of your upper arm on the side of your waist. This will help put your shoulder where it belongs (Step #4). Placing a pillow in front can help prop the arm in place. Your chin is down, and the back of your neck is long. (Step #5)

Make adjustments as necessary to be absolutely comfortable, without undoing the fundamentals of the five basic steps.

Final Tips & Shortcuts

Remind children that skeletons are not just about Halloween and graveyards but that each one of us is a living, breathing skeleton. Encourage them to sense the skeleton that resides deep within themselves and the role it plays in supporting the whole body.

Children love watching the video at http://video.google.com/videoplay?docid=7353579812526357656#. This clever, funny street performance of a skeleton dancing, demonstrates remarkably human movements. After watching the video, you can put on music and pretend that you, too, are dancing skeleton marionettes. During the day, remember as often as you can to "be" a skeleton.

It can be easy to "think" too much about these instructions. Once you grasp the basic concepts, give yourselves over to the puppeteer who pulls the strings attached to the back of your body. Your job is to hang, *relaxed,* from those strings and feel the support that comes from having aligned bones.

Don't expect to "get it" all at once. Work at this slowly and patiently. Remind yourself of your successes, rather than focusing on what is difficult for you. With practice, inhabiting an aligned body will get easier and easier. As you pay attention to yourself, you will become your own best teacher for how to live inside your skin.

Children should be encouraged to remind you when you are not "parking your pelvis" or when you are slouching in front of a computer. They enjoy opportunities to point out our flaws (since we tend to point out so many of theirs), and this will get them thinking and observing more. You can let them that you also have the right to remind them, as well.

Have cushions and wedges available for sitting in cars, at the computer and at the dinner table. Use baby-sized cushions in hammock-style strollers and some baby car seats. * (See Appendix)

Engage in physical play with your children. Not only does active movement offer genuine benefits, it's important for us to model physical activity as something worthwhile that we enjoy doing. Too often, children see us as Mama or Papa Potato, sending the message that life is to be lived on the couch (or sitting in front of a computer for too many hours at a time).

Don't take this—or yourself—too seriously. As important as it is to realign bones for good health, the lessons should never be forced on a child. Keep it fun. If a child is tired or uninterested for any reason, it's best to wait until another time before continuing with the lessons. Just enjoy each other's company!

Shortcut #1 — Going with the Flow

There are any number of ways to visualize and sense your body moving into alignment along the center line. Now that you have learned the basic principles of how different parts of the skeleton relate to each other, here are three short-cuts that offer other ways to put this information together. They are designed to build upon the details you have learned so far. Once you begin to experience a sense for how our human bodies are designed to work, you may discover other benefits, such as feeling *energy* moving through your body. People sometimes report feeling profoundly relaxed and "connected" as they do this, sensing that they are touching a higher state of consciousness. This points to the important role the aligned body plays as a vehicle for conscious living that serves as an anchor to the present moment.

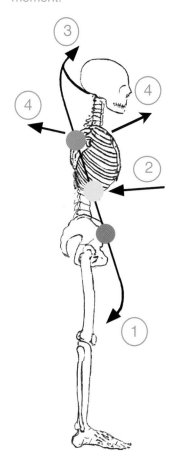

① While standing, find the top rim of the pelvis with your fingers. Let this pelvic rim (red dot) drop forward, as if it were falling to the floor and growing roots behind your heels. This will create maximum distance between your pubic bone and navel (belly button). Notice, too, how the sit bones slide back and widen apart and how the floor of the pelvis opens as you do this. You will recognize this as yet another way to experience "Parking the Pelvis". Establishing your foundation through the pelvis is always a good place to start.

② Imagine the *xiphoid process* (yellow dot) sliding back and up—see Page 69—as if it could actually touch your upper back (green dot). Don't hold your breath, and be sure you are not sucking in your belly. An "action" that you might feel in the belly is good, provided that the pubic bone stays down, away from the navel. This is both Step 2, "Hug a Tree" and Step 3, "Climb a Ladder" put together.

③ As the middle of your back grows wide, it rises up behind you (green dot). The base of your skull also slides up and aims over the top of the head. Remember, keep the *xiphoid process* tucked *back* and *up* at all times (yellow dot).

④ Once the primary anchors are in place—the pelvis and the tethered-in rib cage—the shoulders and front of the chest can open. Trying to open the upper chest without anchoring the bottom of the rib cage first, usually results in arching of the back and compression of the spine. Now, maintaining all of the previous steps, roll your shoulders up, back and *wide*, opening the upper chest by bringing maximum width across its front.

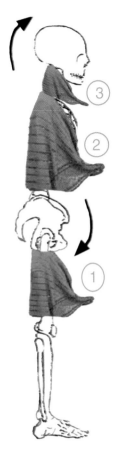

This somewhat peculiar image illustrates another shortcut approach to bringing the skeleton into line with the vertical axis.

① Stand as if holding an imaginary shawl a few inches behind the back of your thighs. (You can use a real shawl at first, if you like.) Move your thighs back until they "touch" the shawl, extending the tailbone out over the top of the shawl. This, of course, is "Park Your Pelvis."

② Hold the shawl, real or imagined, a few inches behind your back and move your back into it, widening your back completely to meet the wrapping shawl. Lift the shawl upwards with your rising shoulder blades and armpits. This is "Hug a Tree" and "Climb a Ladder," respectively.

③ Bring the shawl up to just behind your neck. As with the previous steps, move the back of your neck toward the shawl, taking the time to feel maximum width growing across your neck. The base of the skull will rise up behind you, as the chin drops slightly.

It is important to be especially cautious with this last step, as you don't want to promote any unnecessary tension. It takes time for small muscles in the center of the neck to release. The best way to do this is to "flirt" with the edge of any tension you notice, approaching it delicately and with an emphasis on releasing it with the exhalation. With practice and patience, and a gentle approach, the cervical spine will lengthen over time.

The idea here is to "feel the fullness" of the entire back of your body, while having an equal, symmetrical fullness in the front of the body, as well. This is important in order for the spine to be optimally long, without any compression. Length through the spine is only possible when the lower body—feet, legs and pelvis—are deeply rooted and able to engage with **ground reaction force (GRF)**, the opposite and equal reaction of Newton's Third Law of Motion. This force is not only available through movement, however; it can be called forth at any time, even when sitting or standing still. When we engage with the earth in an active way, we *feel* alive, we have energy available to us. With aligned bones, the channels are open for that energy or "life force" to move through us unimpeded. Along with an ability to relax deeply, these are necessary ingredients to overall good health and well-being, as well as an ability to learn, thrive and meet our full potential. We best serve our children and ourselves when we protect this birthright and promote inhabiting our bodies in this wholly natural way.

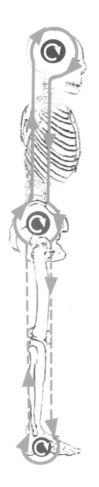

This shortcut is designed to direct the flow of energy through the body, along with the breath, and conveniently works to align the skeleton with the vertical axis at the same time.

Begin by sensing the point at the center of your belly, a couple of inches below your navel and half-way between the front and the back of your abdomen. This is your body's center of gravity, what is known as the *Dan Tien* in Qi Gong and Tai Chi or the *Hara* in Aikido.

Picture a ball located at this center, a ball that is slowly turning forward (red dot). As it turns, it drives the rotation of the pelvis forward, moving the pubic bone down and opening width between the sit bones. *Feel* this inner "engine" at work, if you can.

This approach works equally well whether you are sitting or standing, but if you are standing, this flow can continue down the front of your legs, through the front of your medial arch (blue dot), then turn around under your feet and rise up the back of your legs back up to the pelvis. Here the energy continues upward, but there is no active "lifting" of sit bones, no tensing of any muscles in the buttocks or lower back.

As the flow rises up from the pelvis along the full length of your back and across the back of your neck, you feel the back of your head float upward and your chin drop gently. As the flow of energy now circles forward, following the shape of your skull, it aims inward toward the top of your throat, establishing contact with the length in the neck before turning downward.

Moving down along the front of the torso, the movement of energy re-establishes the forward rotation of the pelvis. This continuous flow of energy through the body is like a wheel that is always turning, regenerating and recycling itself through the body, whenever one puts one's attention to it.

It's easy to coordinate this with the breath by sensing the downward flow of each inhalation through the front of the body and the upward flow of the exhalation through the back. Sense the downward breath anchoring the front of the pelvis into the ground, with the rising breath driving an upward rise through the spine.

Once you've learned how the puppet strings work, these instructions will be easier to understand. The rising up of energy through the back is like having puppet strings gently lifting the back upwards. The forward rotation of the pelvis is the same as having the "Sit Bone Strings" drawn back. The more you learn how to align and relax, the more you will become aware of new and subtle sensations that will contribute to feeling more *alive*! Take time to keep building on these experiences, and encourage the same in your child(ren).

FIVE

Exercises & Helpful Tips
To Help Children & Adults
Stay on Track

The following exercises can all be done while sitting. They are, therefore, easily adapted to a classroom setting and can be interspersed here and there throughout the day's lessons. *It is suggested that parents and teachers become familiar with the finer details of these exercises before teaching them to children.*

Any and all exercises should always be done to conform to basic principles of natural alignment in order to avoid injury or repetitive stress to the body. Adults who understand how to align their bones can play an important role in modeling good alignment and guiding children to this understanding, as well.

Remember that the most useful exercises are ones that simply reinforce the body's natural ways of moving. In this way, a normally active life that includes natural bending, walking, lifting, carrying—even sitting and sleeping in an aligned way—provides the perfect exercise routine.

If you feel pain or strain, it is likely to be an indication that you are doing something incorrectly. Review the details of the Five Puppet String Steps before trying again.

Lengthening the Spine
While Strengthening the "Core"

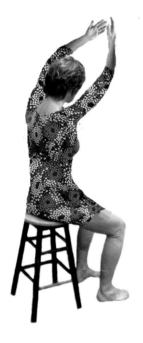

The following simple exercise not only aligns the bones but works to develop the deeper "core" abdominal muscles. Remember to breathe while doing this. Engaging the deeper core muscles keeps the diaphragm elastic, unlike sucking in the belly, which restricts natural breathing.

Sit with your pelvis firmly "parked". Lift your arms overhead, as if reaching for a book on a high shelf out in front of you. Make sure that your breast bone (*sternum*) stays deep inside the chest and doesn't push forward. Wiggle the middle of each armpit up toward the ceiling and make sure that the length you gain in the spine is equal in the back and in the front.

96

Lengthening the Neck

Stabilizing the Shoulders

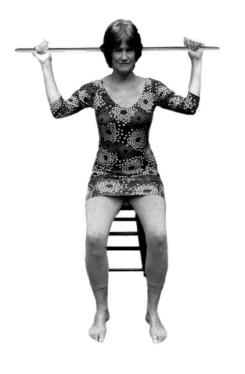

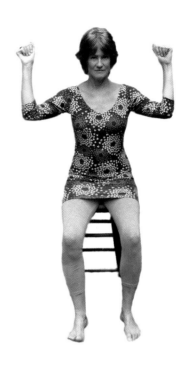

Hold a dowel or stretched scarf behind the base of the skull (at the bottom of the occiput). Drop your chin slightly and gently draw the dowel (or scarf) into the base of the skull and upward, giving a gentle stretch to the back of the neck. This encourages length cervical spine, while reinforcing the action of the puppet string attached at the *occiput*. Be sure there is no straining or striving involved, just a gentle rising within the center of the neck. You can also clasp your hands together at the base of the skull and gently draw the back of the head upward, but using a stick encourages width in the shoulders, as well.

Imagine you are still holding the stick. Begin to draw your elbows forward, as if trying to touch them together. In actuality, your elbows will hardly move at all, since your hands remain in line with your ears, still holding the imaginary stick. You will feel an action in a variety of muscles in and around the shoulders and shoulder blades (*scapulae*). Interestingly, this engages core abdominal muscles. Can you feel them as you do this? You can amplify this by zipping up imaginary jeans from the lowest point in your belly.

Training the Shoulders

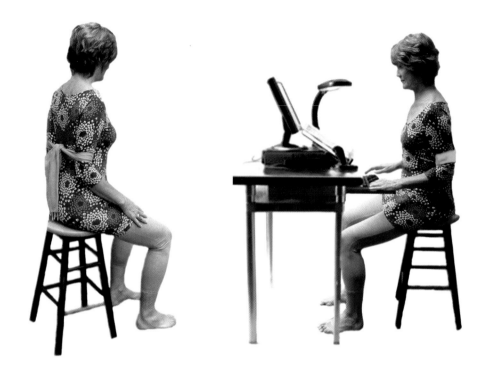

Sitting at the computer for long periods of time can be quite problematic for many people. Discomfort while sitting typically appears in the lower or upper back, across the shoulders and neck. Each of these problems is addressed in the same way, establishing skeletal support from the ground up, first "parking the pelvis" and then lengthening the spine. This way, you are assured that you are supported by aligned bones and that unnecessary muscle tension, most likely the cause of all your misery, will be able to melt away.

Once you've got yourself lined up, per "Puppet Instructions" in Part Two, you might consider tying your elbows behind your back with a scarf or strap.* This will help maintain the placement of the shoulders on top of the rib cage and serve as gentle support of this position.

Be sure in doing this that the strap does not pull your elbows too close together, which will narrow the back and push the chest out in front. Think of your back "meeting" the strap behind you and widening across it. To more deeply engage with the strap, imagine lifting it, and the bottom of the rib cage, up onto a shelf behind you.

* See Appendix for where to order elasticized, adjustable arm bands.

Raising the Arches
& Strengthening the Ankles and Knees

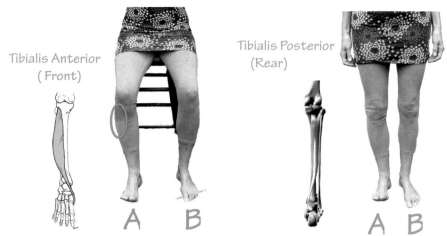

Tibialis Anterior
(Front)

Tibialis Posterior
(Rear)

A   B

A   B

The two *tibialis* muscles attach at the outside of the knee and wrap around the leg, inserting under the primary transverse arch of the foot.. These muscles are weak in people with pronated (rolled in) ankles and flattened arches. Strengthening these muscles stabilizes the ankles and helps keep the arches lifted and buoyant. Many other important foot and leg muscles will re-shape at the same time.

A   Begin by tucking the heels. (Review "Tuck Your Heels" in Part One.). You can do this while sitting by placing your feet 6-8 inches apart, lifting the heels very slightly and turning your knees out. Your toes and the balls of your feet should "grab" at the floor as you bring the outside of the heel onto the floor. Maintain this shape as you lift the toes and ball of one foot up, keeping the heel on the floor. Do this slowly, arching the ball of the foot closer to the heel, as you lift the front of the foot up. Do this until you feel muscles beginning to fatigue but don't overdo it. Repeat on the other side. If you place your hand on your leg in the area of the red oval above, you should be able to feel the action of the *tibialis anterior* muscle working. Now, reverse the action, keeping the ball of the foot in contact with the floor and lifting the *heel* off the floor.

B   Place a pencil on the floor and pick it up with your toes. Once you have the hang of this, do it with only an imaginary pencil, releasing the pencil in front of you as you move forward one tiny step at a time. Keep moving the pencil, real or imaginary, forward on the floor. This exercise strengthens the *tibialis* muscles, anterior and posterior, while working many other muscles in the feet and legs. It also helps train the toes to play a more active role.

Releasing Hamstrings

While most tight muscles will gradually release quite naturally as you learn to realign your bones, focusing on your hamstrings can accelerate your progress in terms of developing the "Happy Dog" rotation of the pelvis. It's helpful to think of a "stretch" as something you *feel* and "releasing tension" as something you *do*. *Stretching, as an activity is often an assault on a muscle instead of establishing the conditions that encourage tension to be released.* Unfortunately, many "hamstring stretches" are done in a way that undermine pelvic rotation or ignore the integrity of a fully lengthened spine.

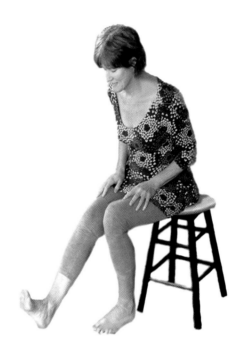

Sit with your feet flat on the floor and your sit bones "parked" on the edge of a chair or stool. Place one foot out in front of you, keeping the knee bent and pressing out through your heel as your toes aim back toward you. Move your heel away from you. If you begin to feel a stretching sensation in the back of your thigh, pause there, and bring your attention to your breath.

Breathing is the key to releasing tension. Imagine the inhaling breath actually touching the place(s) where you are feeling a stretch, and then, as you exhale, sense the tension in your muscle(s) melting away. If you find this difficult, you may have stretched too far. Try easing up somewhat, so that you are simply "flirting" with the sensations.

If, on the other hand, you are able to fully extend your leg without feeling much sensation at all, begin to fold forward at the hips, keeping the fullness in your back and the length in your spine and proceed as above.

The flexibility gained from "stretching" will only last as long as the exercises are repeated regularly. Genuine, lasting flexibility (meaning muscles that have balanced tonus, or elasticity) is the natural outcome of muscles being attached to aligned bones.

Bend, Bend and Bend Some More

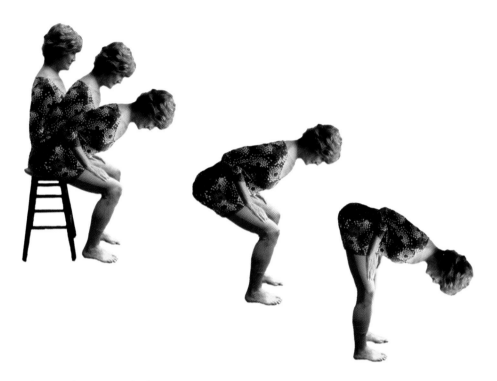

The sit bones slide back and the knees bend wide to initiate all bending movements. The spine and torso remain straight. When getting up from a chair, draw your feet in closer to you and let the sit bones slide out behind you until your weight is on your feet. Push your feet into the floor to bring yourself up. Your chin remains slightly dropped, and the back of neck is long throughout. Bend to pick things up off the floor many times a day. Scatter pennies across the floor and pick them up one at a time. Involve yourself in activities, such as gardening, that require frequent bending. Put on music and bend to the beat. You'll never have to go to the gym, if you do this. Just make sure your sit bones remain as far apart as possible in all that you do.

Bending naturally does it all—it lifts the arches, strengthens and stabilizes the primary, weight-bearing joints (ankles, knees and hips), keeps the hamstrings lengthened, and conditions the natural strength of leg muscles. It teaches us how to move according to our natural biomechanical design, while promoting genuine, easy flexibility. It trains the body to rely on the legs to move us through space, rather than unnecessary, spine-shortening action in muscles above the hips.

BIBLIOGRAPHY

Although there is currently great interest in matters related to children's health, there is very little information on the relationship of "posture" to children's overall health and how it affects their sense of wellbeing, as well as their ability to study and learn. Even research by some of the most prestigious institutions continues to remain largely irrelevant, because of the widespread misunderstanding of how a natural human body actually works.

American Pain Society. *Pediatric Chronic Pain: Significance of the Problem;* Position Statement; http://www.ampainsoc.org/advocacy/pediatric.htm

Balague F et al. *Low-back pain in school children: An epidemiological study.* Scandinavian Journal of Rehabilitative Medicine, 1988, Vol 20, 175-179.

Children's Hospital Boston. Harvard Medical School. *Sports Injury Statistics; 2007*

Goldthwait, J., M.D.; Brown, L., M.D.; Swaim, L.,M.D.; Kuhns, J., M.D., and Kerr, W., M.D. *Essentials of Body Mechanics in Health and Disease,* Philadelphia: J. B. Lippincott Company, 1934.

Junnila, J., Cartwright, V. *Chronic Musculoskeletal Pain in Children: Part I. Initial Evaluation.* American Family Physician, 2006.

Kratenova, J; Zejglicova, K; Maly, M; Filipova, V. *Prevalence and risk factors of poor posture in school children in the Czech Republic.* Journal of School Health, 2007.

Matthew, A. *Implications for Education in the Work of F.M. Alexander.* Thesis - An Exploratory Project in a Public School Classroom; 1984.

Monson, N.; Wisoff, D. *Children and Posture: Why it Really Matters.* http://denver.yourhub.com/Lafayette/Stories/Archive/Health-Fitness/Resources/Story~385997.aspx

Olsen T et al. *The epidemiology of low-back pain in an adolescent population.* American Journal of Emergency Medicine, May 1994, Vol 12(3), 334-336.

Pediatrics / Children's Health. *Children Carrying Heavy Backpacks Risk Poor Posture, Injury* http://www.medicalnewstoday.com/articles/25106.php

Roodenburg, Herman. *How to Sit, Stand or Walk: Toward a Historical Anthropology of Dutch Paintings". In Looking at Seventeenth-Century Dutch Art: Realism Reconsidered, ed.* Wayne Franits. New York: Cambridge University Press.1997.

Schneider, I. *Balance, Posture and Movement: Optimizing Children's Learning Capacities Through Integration of the Sensory Motor System.* Assoc. of Waldorf Schools of North America, 2001.

Smithsonian Institution, *Human Origins Project* http://anthropology.si.edu/humanorigins/ha/sap.htm

Triano, J.J. *Backpacks and Back Pain in Children,* Spine Health; http://www.spine-health.com/conditions/back-pain/backpacks-and-back-pain-children; 200

Troussler B et al. *Back pain in school children: A study among 1178 pupils.* Scandinavian Journal of Rehabilitative Medicine, 1994, Vol 26, 143-146.

Volinn E. *The epidemiology of low back pain in the rest of the world. A review of surveys in low middle-income countries.* Spine 1997 Aug 1;22(15):1747-54.

ACKNOWLEDGEMENTS

Many people have contributed in helping to bring this book to fruition, from its earliest inception to its final outcome. None of this, of course, would ever have been possible without the pioneering work of Noelle Perez, Jean Couch and others who have continuously dedicated themselves to bringing these ideas forward. I have been most fortunate to benefit from the inspiration, participation, professional support, encouragement and friendship of many people. I would like to make special acknowledgement of Ren Scott, Grace Peyerwold, Irene McNeely, Kathryn Grout, Thea Beckett, Carter Beckett, Patra Conley, Camille Scofield, Hettie Scofield, Kathy Wines, Kaholo Deguman, Anne Marie Claire, Rhona Klein, Tracey Nicholas, John Metcalf, Peggy O'Mara, Christiane Northrup, Moline Whitson, Barry Siegel, Sherry Genauer, Gabe Genauer, Talia Genauer, Jay Genauer, Owen Nguyen, Betty Lee, Tabor Bergh, Stacey Tripeny, Billy Sammons, Joanna Hunter, Paul Burt, Ginny Weissman, Min Gates, Mary Copenlaver, Coease Scott, Nina Scott, Maria Peyerwold, Cindy Debus, Jan Cooper, Kenneth Lahti, Patricia Salmon, Sally Mermel, Dianne Horwitz, Dawn Pung, Wendy Miyamoto, Linda Haynes, Marisa Miyashiro, Patti Chikasuye, Diane Li, Milo Jarvis, Marianne Kuipers-Tilanus, Ho-Sheng Chi, Steve Rayne, Fiona Rayne, Ellery Rayne, Jill Schatten, John Andrew, Vicki Lind, Peg Warren, Bonnie McAnnis, Brian Duby, Daniel Ryan, Lauren Kamp, Kevin Chambers, Josh Leake, and Alyssa O'Banion.

Mahalo to my beautiful, wonderful family—Meredith, Kendra, Evan, Wendell, Weston, Evan B, Precious, Alika, Leslie, Kristin, Jack, Owen, and everyone else in the ever-growing Porter/Ing 'Ohana. An extra special thank you goes to Evan Ing for his enthusiastic and talented technical support and to Kathryn Grout for generous editing help.

I have created most of the illustrations in this book, as well as having produced the layout. Any errors or inaccuracies in the presentation of this information are mine alone.

PHOTO CREDITS

Thank you to the following for kindly allowing the use of their photographs:

Jack Nguyen

Magnus Franklin

Tara Bruce

Francis Irving

Monica Misiowiec

Sumati Kathrine Brekke

Mary Goodrich   www.marygoodrich.com

United States Library of Congress

iStock.com

Wikimedia.org

APPENDIX

Visit NaturalPostureSolutions.com to learn about effective and affordable support products for babies, teens and adults.

Classroom Seating

Appropriate classroom desk chairs are almost non-existent, even among those companies that advertise "ergonomic" chairs for students. Child-sized wedge-shaped cushions* can be used with existing chairs to "park the pelvis". Such cushions convert those chairs force a tucked pelvis, into providing support for a naturally tilted pelvis. Such cushions are an inexpensive alternative, even for school districts with budgetary limitations. The Wedge, available at NaturalPostureSolutions.com is made out of non-skid material and works well on any surface, including wood or plastic.

Some innovative schools have been doing away with desk chairs altogether and have been incorporating large "therapy" balls in their place. The use of these balls has shown positive results, most especially with children who have been diagnosed with ADHD (http://www.ateachabout.com/pdf/ClassroomSeatingUsingBalls.pdf) because the balls offer students an opportunity for dynamic movement throughout the day. It is still possible to sit poorly on a ball, so learning how to "park the pelvis" is important. A good selection of child-size balls is available at wittfitt.com, along with additional information. Both sitting wedges and balls are economical solutions for schools with limited budgets.

Teachers have many opportunities each day to include information from this book in their students' curriculum. What more important information is there than helping children learn how to live in relaxed, comfortable bodies that will serve them with good health throughout their entire lives?

At-Home Seating

Parents can help their children by providing them with the tools they need for sitting upright in a natural, comfortable way. (Visit NaturalPostureSolutions.com and babywedgie.com.)* Parents of infants can inform themselves about natural alignment, so as to protect their babies and toddlers from losing their it in the first place. Babies' feet should be put in shoes as seldom as possible, so as to let the toes and arches develop natural strength and ways of moving. When shoes are worn, they should have soft soles and plenty of room for the feet to move within the shoe box. Wearing shoes with hard soles may be necessary, in certain situations, but should not be relied upon, as a rule.

Parents can discuss with their children the importance of remaining aligned, sharing the concepts in this book and giving children the tools they need for maintaining this alignment in as many situations as possible. Towels and small fleece blankets can be folded into wedge-shaped cushions, or wedge-shaped cushions can be purchased. (NaturalPostureSolutions.com.) Most important of all, parents need to model good posture for their children, whenever possible. The benefits of this are two-fold: Not only will you be protecting your child's future health, you'll be protecting your own, as well!

Such products have not been tested by the National Highway Traffic Safety Administration and, therefore, can not be recommended for use in car seats.

TEACHERS OF NATURAL ALIGNMENT

The following is a partial list of people who teach the principles of natural alignment under various names. No matter what the method is called, it must be based, thoroughly and completely, on the natural biomechanical design that is inherent to the human species. Anything other than this, while it may offer certain benefits, does not meet the criteria for "natural alignment".

New insights about the universal features of natural human design have been coming to light in recent years, thanks in large part to Noelle Perez who first brought attention to these concepts. Since the 1990s, information about how the body *really* works has continued to grow and new ways to teach this to others have continued to be developed. The "Puppet Posture" and "Sad Dog, Happy Dog" concepts have been developed by Kathleen Porter and are not taught by anyone else at this time. Different teachers bring their own unique insights and talents to sharing this, contributing to a growing body of work and influence to this developing field. No distinction is made here between the effectiveness or value of these differing approaches, as one method may be more easily understood and integrated by one person than another. The intention in making this list available is to provide opportunities for learning natural alignment to as many people in as many places as possible. Please contact me if your name should be included on this this list. kathleen@naturalalignment.com

Noelle Perez and teachers
affiliated with
L'Institut Superieur d'Aplomb
www.isaplomb.org
Paris, France

Jean Couch and teachers
affiliated with The Balance Center
650-856-2000
jean@balancecenter.com
Palo Alto, CA

Kathleen Porter
503-505-1996
kathleen@naturalalignment.com
Portland, OR

Dana Davis
707-658-2599
dana@sonomabodybalance.com
Petaluma, CA

Jean Farmwald
650-787-8781
jfarmwald@earthlink.net
Palo Alto, CA

Kay Hackney
907-457-1481
mkhackney@acsalaska.net
Fairbanks, AK

Mary Sinclair
614-906-0260
balancemares@netzero.net
Columbus, OH

Barbara Wilkens
650/494-7630
barbannwilkens@gmail.com
Palo Alto, CA

Karen Werner
206-579-0205
karenlee29@comcast.net
Federal Way, WA

Thea Sawyer
408-489-9436
thea@liveinbalance.com
San Jose, CA

Lauri Moschini
650-269-4875
laurimoschini@yahoo.com
Mountain View, CA

Kim Thompson
301-519-9532
kim@optimizedmovement. com
Gaithersburg, MD

Margaret Gilday
610-388-1624
margaretgilday@live.com
Cadds Ford, PA

Jay Bunker
510/213-0546
jaybunker@earthlink.net
Albany, CA

Sukha Carfagno
650/399-6753
roquena.lahonda@
sbcglobal.net
La Honda, CA

Nora Braverman
646-784-0748
nvbpt@yahoo.com
New York, NY

Esther Gokhale
650-324-3244
info@egwellness.com
Palo Alto, CA

Angelika Thusius
541-552-0992
Ashland, OR

Lisa Ann McCall
214.328.8400
lisaann@mccallmethod.com
Dallas, TX

Visit NaturalPostureSolutions.com to learn about:

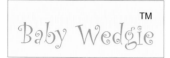

Baby-size cushion that protects a baby's spine in strollers and other sitting devices. Buckwheat filled, non-skid fabric. Promotes and supports baby's natural alignment.

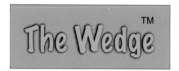

Mini-wedge cushion that "parks the pelvis" and supports the spine in many sitting situations. Ideal for school-age children, teen and adults. Small and portable. Keep one at your desk, one in your car, one in your bag. Makes a great gift.

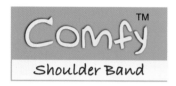

Plush elastic support for comfortable, relaxed shoulders while working at a computer or other sitting tasks. Use this adjustable, elasticized strap to help "train" the shoulders to rest on top of the rib cage where they belong. Brings instant relief to tight, aching shoulder muscles.

Books by Kathleen Porter: Available at NaturalPostureSolutions.com as well as book stores and other book sellers

Ageless Spine, Lasting Health:
The Open Secret to Pain-free Living
and Comfortable Aging
(Synergy, 2006)
$24.95

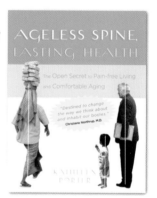

"Kathleen Porter's insights about skeletal alignment are destined to change the way we think about and inhabit our bodies."

Christiane Northrup, M.D.

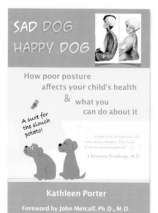

Sad Dog, Happy Dog:
How Poor Posture Affects Children's Health
And What to Do About It
(Mekevan Press, 2010)
$24.95